LON106

W 20

Educating the Future GP

The Course Organizer's Handbook

SECOND EDITION

Patrick McEvoy

Radcliffe Medical Press

© 1998 Patrick McEvoy

Radcliffe Medical Press Ltd
18 Marcham Road, Abingdon, Oxon OX14 1AA, UK

First edition 1993

Reprinted 2006

British Library Cataloguing in Publication Data

A catalogue record for this book is available from the British Library.

ISBN 1 85775 281 3

Library of Congress Cataloging-in-Publication Data is available.

Typeset by Advance Typesetting Ltd, Oxon
Printed and bound in Great Britain by TJI Digital, Padstow, Cornwall

Contents

Foreword

From its early years the Association of Course Organizers recognized the need for a handbook principally to act as a guide for new course organizers. We imagined that such a publication might simply consist of a few loose-leaf sheets containing useful addresses, a bibliography and general advice. It was therefore with some surprise and much delight that course organizers greeted the first edition of this book in 1993. Paddy McEvoy was not content to follow the simple brief we had envisaged. Instead he showed immense creativity and hard work by producing a book which covered the whole range of GP training. Not only that but a book that was both eminently readable and an essential work of reference. Paddy illuminated the work of the course organizer with scholarship, imagination and humour. Perhaps his greatest skill was to capture in the book the varied emotions of course organizers.

Writing a second edition could have been a great anticlimax. After all, perhaps the most significant happening in vocational training in Britain since the first edition has been the advent of compulsory summative assessment – hardly a very exciting event to write about. You will indeed find a guide to summative assessment in this book but you will also find that Paddy's creativity is still in top gear. As well as updating and revising the book throughout there are new chapters which show that insularity is not for Paddy – and should not be for us. With many European GP registrars choosing to train in this country we have a great deal to learn from their cultures and systems. GP registrars obviously need to be familiar with many other cultures as well. Paddy has managed to include chapters about the wider context of training without making the book overly long or losing any of the delightful flavour of the first edition.

As someone just starting for a second time as a course organizer, I feel this book will act both as a security blanket for me and as a spur to creativity. It may do other things for you but I have no doubt that you will find it both useful and enjoyable.

Paul Sackin
Former secretary, ACO
April 1998

Preface

'To be trained is to arrive; to be educated is to continue to travel'
(Kenneth Calman, *The Profession of Medicine*)

Something happened to general practice in the UK in the 1990s. It is called change. When this book was commissioned by the Association of Course Organizers in 1990 there was the feeling that our collective experience should be collated and circulated to the membership so that new and isolated course organizers could find a fast track to carrying out a well-developed role. When a revisit became necessary it was clear that so much was changing that nothing short of total revision would suffice.

For GPs the decade has brought a new contract, accelerated evolution of the job description, inversion of the commissioning pyramid in the NHS, manpower shortage and increasing influences from continental Europe. There is evidence of a crisis of identity among GPs with, perhaps, a cautious optimism about the future.

It would be remarkable if this fluid state were not reflected in the training process, or reflected on by the teachers. Recent developments include assessment, the certification process, regulatory framework, structure of the regional educational team and the organization and delivery of medical education from university entrance to retirement. Development has not been limited to these administrative areas. There are genuinely new educational approaches such as problem-based and portfolio-based learning, multiprofessionalism, an emphasis on evidence-based thinking and information technology and a fresh awareness of the need to develop the academic base of primary care.

Reactions to the first edition taught me a great deal. I learnt that the body of knowledge which is relevant to course organizers is also vital to the trainers and teachers of all health care professionals. Whether in the UK and Ireland, in Europe and abroad, at graduate or undergraduate level, it seems we plough a common field of educational theory and practice, group work and management, despite our various systems of care. It was intriguing to find that these themes are also finding their way into the everyday work of general practitioners and 'the team'. I hope that this book will continue to be of service to course organizers and that it will also be of interest to this wider constituency.

Thus, the scope of *Educating the Future GP* has had to be expanded. Additional chapters acknowledge the place of vocational training as a transitional phase linking undergraduate and continuing medical education, and reflect the changes in the examination system and the transnational influences which are likely to impinge increasingly on training for primary care into the millennium and beyond.

Assistance from many sources shaped the first edition. I reiterate my thanks to those acknowledged herein. I have had to revisit many of them as well as tap new sources.

Patrick McEvoy
April 1998

Acknowledgements

My thanks go firstly to my wife, Hazel, whose doctoral thesis on adult education greatly informed the chapters on education; to my children, Siobhan, Frances, Mark and John who may have felt that they had lost a father for weeks at a time; the many course organizers on whose conversations I eavesdropped; the ACO Executive for commissioning this book – its members, past and present, have been unfailingly supportive; the staff of the Information Department of the Royal College of General Practitioners and to representatives of the various organizations described in Chapter 16.

I thank the following friends and colleagues who contributed in various ways. Drs John Salinsky, Paul Sackin, Paul Wright and Shake Siegel for vetting parts of the text; Frank O'Deorain and staff at the medical library at Altnagelvin Area Hospital; Esme O'Brien, Siobhan Kelly and Debora Donaghy for secretarial services; Neil Doherty, Bill Boyle and Joe O'Reilly for proofreading and technical assistance. I gratefully acknowledge the help and interest shown by my partners at the Aberfoyle Medical Practice, Derry and by colleagues in the Northern Ireland Vocational Training Scheme. In particular, my senior partner Dr Peter Fallon who introduced me to training and course organizing and has been a mentor to me on the journey.

There is no better metaphor for education for general practice than that of a journey and its course has been enlivened for me for 13 years by the company of those essential fellow travellers – the registrars in general practice training. This book owes much to them.

A final acknowledgement of debt and esteem goes to an eminent pilgrim on the way of education for general practice. Eric Gambril did me the honour of offering to write the Foreword. Sadly, he did not live to fulfil this promise.

Patrick McEvoy
April 1998

I dedicate this book to my wife, Hazel, my children, Siobhan, Frances, Mark and John and all my fellow course organizers

Part 1

First steps

Overview

These opening chapters offer a bird's-eye view of course organizing by skimming over the details and highlighting the main features of the terrain.

I know someone who was bitterly disappointed after a holiday in East Africa because he was unable to take a photograph of Mount Kilimanjaro. Most of the time it was shrouded in mist (at least the interesting bits were), and on the one clear day he had to drive so far back, to get both ends into the frame, that it lacked grandeur. An alternative might have been to paint it, employing a bit of artistic licence, leaving in the clouds around the base but accentuating the lofty, shimmering peaks and throwing in a few wild animals in the foreground to provide life and a sense of depth.

Our equivalent of the 'wild animals' are the scenarios, which provide perspective on the scene. The main features which are highlighted include an account of a survey of the needs of course organizers (Chapter 1), a package of hints on getting started (Chapter 2) and an attempt to define the work and identity of the course organizer (Chapter 3).

Unfamiliar themes and terminology in these chapters will be more fully explored in the remaining Parts – like zooming in on bits of Kilimanjaro. The broad base of the mountain should then gradually emerge from the clouds.

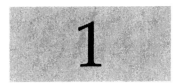

1

The needs of new course organizers

Introduction

In an attempt to discover the needs of new course organizers, a survey was carried out at a conference of the Association of Course Organizers (McEvoy, 1993). Participants were asked to fill in a questionnaire about the anxieties and needs they had experienced in the early phase of their work as course organizers, and to indicate what they had found helpful at that time.

Although many of the responses appear to emphasize the negative aspects of course organizing, they did provide a framework of suggestions which could make the start-up period smoother than it might otherwise be.

Responses were received from 40 course organizers – some new, some very experienced – representing 20 regions of the UK. Respondents were particularly concerned about:

- lack of educational qualifications
- lack of qualifications in administration and management
- vagueness of job descriptions
- lack of knowledge about the organizational framework
- the need for supportive structures
- the need for communication skills, especially in group work.

A few quotations put a human face on this:

- *'The principal problem when I was new to course organization was coping with an enormous, open-ended list of tasks which were unidentifiable until a crisis occurred'*
- *'Will I be able to do it and cope with the stresses involved?'*
- *'Being a single-handed course organizer I have no-one to share problems with. I don't know how I'm doing. Is it okay?'*

- *'I have found that meeting other course organizers in a semi-social, semi-educational way (such as this conference), has done wonders for my confidence'*
- *'I need organizational skills – running a flexible course can cause a lot of headaches'*
- *'I am not properly trained in educational and group skills'*
- *'I want to help SHOs and stressed trainees'*
- *'The job description should be simpler'*
- *'Course organizing conflicts with my practice and home life'*
- *'I lack influence in the hospital training posts'*
- *'I need a reliable secretary'.*

Far from being a source of dismay, it may be comforting to the new course organizer to know the extent to which other professionals share anxieties about self-esteem and their teaching skills, and struggle to make sense of the curriculum, the structures and the job description.

The important outcome – identifying what could have helped – can be summarized in the following recommendations.

1 New or aspiring course organizers should be funded to attend courses in which the job's nature, aims and methods are explored. They should be encouraged to visit other vocational training schemes as observers.
2 After being appointed they need a period of apprenticeship with an experienced mentor, and regular opportunities to meet their peers at the local, regional and national level to learn about the structure of vocational training, to ventilate feeling and to explore problems.
3 Particular training is needed in teaching, communication, counselling, group work, assessment and management skills.
4 The job description and regional lines of communication should be as explicit and simple as possible, although it should be recognized that, with growing experience, the new course organizer will soon feel comfortable with a wider range of activities and responsibilities.
5 Adequate resources should be provided. The minimum provision should be reliable secretarial assistance and a mentor, i.e. an experienced course organizer who can provide initial and continuing support, even if intermittently or from a distance.

This handbook is a response to the expressed needs of the course organizer in his or her early days. It is hoped that it will provoke as many questions as it addresses and that it will be re-edited by each owner to suit the individual situation and needs, with additions, inserts and appropriate deletions. It does not aspire to be a textbook for all course organizers everywhere – the range of possibilities is too wide for that. The chief danger of this book is that its focus on areas of challenge and difficulty in course organizing may obscure the reward of a stimulating, satisfying and engrossing role in the formation of a generation of new colleagues in the most rapidly evolving area of the medical profession – the provision of primary health care to the people of these islands.

Scenario: The doctor's dilemma: what sort of course organizer?

Act I: Exploring

Dr Meeke, a trainer, talks to Dr Best, a retiring course organizer.

Meeke: *Okay. So if course organizing is undervalued, time consuming and hard work, why do you do it?*

Best: *I've often asked myself that. The only other person who asks me that is my wife ... apart from other course organizers that is.*

Meeke: *There must be something in it for you, but all we hear about from course organizers is complaints and agitation for more resources.*

Best: *That's a bit unfair! We also agitate for less work! Unfortunately most GPs, even trainers, don't know much about what course organizers do. At least the GMSC and the RCGP agreed that we should get paid better – and it took a lot of shouting to get even that! Little else about course organizers gets into print in the medical magazines.*

Meeke: *Well, I've seen a few things in print. For instance, why is there such a shortage of applicants? Why do most course organizers stick the job for less than five years? And why do partners of course organizers complain that they're always away? It sounds like a mess. You've either got an image problem or some kind of identity problem.*

Best: *Nonsense! The shortage of applicants is relative. The job is an unknown quantity to most people. GPs tend to be patient centred and they've been busy enough since the 1990 contract and all the administrative things they do. Mostly it's only open to trainers and a trainer may have difficulty doing both. The pay doesn't compensate a practice for losing a partner for two sessions a week. It's not merely an image problem, there are real disincentives. It takes a fair degree of commitment on the part of the course organizer and his partners to make it work.*

Meeke: *Is it an escape from being a GP?*

Best: *You can't escape from being a GP, and that can be a problem in itself. Many GPs feel a real need for new challenges, because there's not much of a career ladder once you're in.*

Meeke: *So watch out for the mid-life crisis!*

Best: *Well, a real part of professional development is related to goals, achievements and making sense of what we do. This leads many GPs into a teaching role. A doctor's commitment to teaching is enshrined in things as basic as his title (which means 'teacher') and the Hippocratic Oath about 'passing on this knowledge'. General practice is a growth area now, and it's gaining respect within the profession. To be an educator in a vital area of medicine is a high-status activity.*

Meeke: *Status implies recognition – by whom?*

Best: *GPs have always had a position of status in the community, but they've always been undervalued by the hospital establishment. GP educators are a relatively new breed.*

No-one can talk you into becoming a course organizer. Do it only if you feel that you'd enjoy the weekly meeting with a group of young doctors... I'm always learning about myself and my practice. I get paid to keep up to date, which I would have to do somehow in any case. Why don't you spend a few minutes writing down your own feelings and thoughts about why you're a trainer, what you get out of it, and what makes you curious about course organizing?

Exercise 1	
Why am I a trainer	Why be a course organizer?

Act II: The interview: to appoint or disappoint?

(Dr Meeke enters and takes his seat in front of the horseshoe-shaped desk)

Dean: *Thank you for coming to be interviewed for one of the course organizer vacancies in our Region. As you no doubt know, I'm in charge of all postgraduate education for the Region. Your first questioner will be Dr Smartt, Regional Director in general practice. Then Dr Keen, an experienced course organizer, will take things a bit further.*

Smartt: *Good morning Dr Meeke. So you want to be a course organizer, good show! Would you like to tell me a bit about yourself and why you applied?*

Meeke: *Well... I've been in practice for 10 years. It's a suburban training practice and I've been a trainer for four or five years. I've always enjoyed teaching, and I thought it was time for a new challenge. The local course organizer was a very good chap and before his retirement he encouraged me to get involved in the day-release course. I began to find that more interesting than one-to-one teaching in the practice. Since he went off I've been helping to keep things going. I've learned a lot, sitting in on the sessions he arranged. I've had a lot of encouragement from the other local trainers to apply for the vacancy. I also think it would make me a better GP – new ideas, keeping up to date, that sort of thing.*

Smartt: *Splendid! And what about your experience in education?*

Meeke: *Apart from the training in one-to-one teaching I had as a trainer and giving a talk or two each year to the day-release course... I've given classes for Red Cross volunteers and had the occasional medical student attached. I've always enjoyed talking about my work and keep myself reasonably up to date.*

Smartt: *Have you any experience of groups?*

Meeke: *I was scout leader at school and ran a folk group at college. I like talking to groups. Besides, I work in a group practice. That can be quite a challenging group!*

Smartt: *Yes, yes, very good. What about publications?*

Meeke: *No... Not really, so far, but I've done a few audits.*

Smartt: *Thank you Dr Meeke. I'll hand you over to Dr Keen.*

Keen: *Dr Meeke, what do your colleagues in the practice think about your plans to be a course organizer?*

Meeke: *Oh, they're all for it, provided it doesn't take me away from practice and I do it in my own time. One of them did mention that a session or two at the British Chemicals plant might be more convenient from the practice point of view but I don't think he really meant it.*

Keen: *Tell me about your educational philosophy, Dr Meeke.*

Meeke: *Um... I'm not sure I...*

Keen: *Not to worry. What are your thoughts on the place of appraisal in vocational training?*

Meeke: *Well, appraisal is a very important part of formative assessment – Manchester Scales and all that. I've never had any difficulty with my trainees. We have the odd chat about their progress, and they have always passed the College exam.*

Keen: *What do you think of the contribution of the hospital consultants to vocational training?*

Meeke: *I hear they give good lectures at the release course. Always ready to oblige and very helpful on the whole.*

Keen: *Thank you, Dr Meeke. I'll hand you back to the chairman.*

Dean: *Perhaps there are questions you would like to ask us at this point?*

Meeke: *One or two. I've always had a trainee in my practice, they make a great contribution. There won't be any problem about continuing...?*

Dean: *Um... I'll ask Dr Smartt to answer that.*

Smartt: *Yes indeed! Very good question. Let me put it this way. Since the trainee is supernumerary, I'm sure your practice would not have any problem in continuing without one. You'll be busy enough without having to be both course organizer and trainer. Couldn't expect you to do both. We don't encourage it in this Region. Now perhaps if one of your partners applied to become trainer, after a while – well, you never know.*

Meeke: *But I've committed myself to taking on a trainee for this year! I don't feel I can let her down.*

Dean: *Under the circumstances, yes, you do have the right to do both. But I would think carefully about that, if I were you. Both make heavy demands. So you can fulfil your obligations to this trainee even if we appoint you as course organizer. Any other questions?*

Meeke: *Yes – what training and support will I receive if I am appointed?*

Dean: *Let me assure you that Dr Smartt and his associates would support you all the way! Any problems, just phone them. About training, the Association of Course Organizers run something every year don't they, Dr Keen.*

Keen: *Yes indeed. Don't worry about that, though; most new course organizers pick up the job as they go along quite well.*

Dean: *Thank you for coming along Dr Meeke. We'll be in touch. Good morning.*

(Exit Meeke stage left)

Dean: *Well, gentlemen, what do you think? Dr Keen?*

Keen: *He didn't seem to know a lot about groups and he wasn't strong on educational theory and I'm not sure he has the backing he'll need from his practice – those hints about not taking time out and going for sessions in industry leave me wondering. I have reservations.*

Dean: *Come, come, Dr Keen... What about Pendleton's rule? Positives first. Smartt?*

Smartt: *Well, Dr Dean. He did okay as a trainer and he had some idea about appraisal; sound practice; he enjoys teaching. I like him. Good chap. One of his partners is in line to be a trainer, so the practice will cope. He's not too clear about what the job entails, but neither were we at his stage – until we started doing it. I think he'll get on all right, Dean.*

Dean: *Now Keen, any further thoughts?*

Keen: *I would like to see how he compares with the others. Who's the next candidate, Dean?*

Dean: *Mmmm... there isn't one. Mind you, we had a couple of enquiries and one other application, but he withdrew. Can't think why. No, I think Dr Meeke will do nicely. He's got potential. I propose we appoint him. I expect you'll show him the ropes, Keen. I think we have a decision. Time for coffee?*

Interlude: A letter from the Regional Director

Dear Dr Meeke

Congratulations. Your application has been successful. You are appointed as Course Organizer with responsibility for the district day-release course from 1 August.

This is a position of great responsibility...

(Meeke: Does he mean 'don't screw up?')

... and status within the profession.

(Meeke: Recognized by the millions who know what a course organizer is!)

A few guidelines about the job may help you initially. I enclose the regional statement of aims for vocational training. Within limits, you will have a lot of autonomy. I have asked Dr Smartt to see you from time to time to discuss progress. However you will have to be self-directed.

(Meeke: Does he mean isolated and under-resourced?)

... self learning

(Meeke: I think this means 'learn on the job')

... multifaceted

(Meeke: Which means there is no clear job description but lots of jobs to do)
   ... and flexible.
(Meeke: Which means much the same)
   Finally, if you have any problems, contact Dr Keen.

   Yours sincerely

   W J Smartt
   Regional Adviser

Act III: Party time

Meeke: *Good news, I've just been appointed a course organizer.*
Mrs Glass: *Congratulations! What's a course organizer?*
Meeke: *It's someone who teaches general practice to young doctors.*
Mrs Glass: *Oh, my husband's a trainer too.*
Meeke: *Well, they're a bit different. A course organizer runs classes for groups of trainees on a day-release course.*
Mrs Glass: *So you're going to be a real teacher just like me, have your own classroom and all that?*
Meeke: *Something like that.*
Mrs Glass: *I suppose it'll be a relief to be away from the surgery, not to have to get out of bed at night and so forth.*
Meeke: *No, that has to go on, I don't quit being a GP. I do this extra.*
Mrs Glass: *Will you be going off somewhere to train before you get teaching, or do you take night classes?*
Meeke: *Well, no. I just start holding my course next month.*
Mrs Glass: *That's quick. So how do you become a GP teacher?*
Meeke: *I'll go to the odd conference, do a bit of reading; that sort of thing.*
Mrs Glass: *And that will make you a teacher? That's not fair.*
Meeke: *Why not?*
Mrs Glass: *Well, I'm a teacher. I spent three years training to be a teacher, had a probationary year, worked for a few years. Now I'm doing a DAISE; there's a lot to it.*
Meeke: *What's a DAISE?*
Mrs Glass: *It's a Diploma in Advanced Studies in Education – takes one year full-time at University or two years part-time. I'm learning a lot and there's always so much more. But I'm curious about this. You'll be teaching doctors to be GPs. So what qualifications in teaching will you need? It's taken me five years to learn about teaching. It doesn't seem fair that you can do it in a few weekends. Not fair to the students, I mean.*
Meeke: *It's always been like that in medicine. Can I get you another drink?*
(Exit hurriedly)

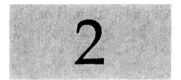

2

Starting up

Scenario: A letter from a retiring course organizer

Dear John

Congratulations course organizer! Smartt phoned me after the interview and said you might be in touch. He asked me to give you some support until you 'find your feet'. I got your letter just as I'm about to go on holiday. I'm not surprised that you don't know where to start. I must say, I got that feeling every August as the start of each year loomed up.

I enclose a few pages of notes which I threw together some time ago for the ACO and came across it again just as I was packing up, so you can be getting on with things. Hope you don't mind distance learning – there's a lot of it in course organizing. We'll arrange a few sessions to talk things over face-to-face when I get back. I'm sure you'll have a few issues to raise and, as I face life without course organizing, I'll quite enjoy getting it out of my system ('de-roling' and all that – the jargon becomes part of you after a while. Maybe that will wear off too!).

See you soon and meantime remember one thing – have fun, make it fun.

Ronnie Best

Introduction

Starting up as a new course organizer is a time of crisis and challenge. It is tempting to focus on the problems once the first glow of success has faded. It is important to recognize that course organizers are being increasingly appreciated and valued as innovators within medical education. Even if you work in relative isolation, you are joining a regional team of people who are enthusiastic about the process of equipping young doctors for the most rapidly developing area of medicine. This involves critical appraisal of the job of general practice and the systems which govern it. Much of the negativity you may encounter reflects a deep concern that general practice education should be properly esteemed, properly resourced and effectively carried out.

Ultimately it is a question of self-esteem. If you believe that the task has considerable status and value you will find that apprehensions reflect a sense of purpose, and difficulties become challenges.

What is a day-release course for?

Before you start wondering what you are going to do on the course you might ask yourself why it exists. This may be sailing perilously close to questioning the need for course organizers. The reasons behind our model of vocational training, based on lots of hospital work and apprenticeship to a trainer with day-release training, is only worth exploring at this point if you want a topic for a MD thesis. It is sufficient for now to say that ours is only one of many existing models of training. For example, in Belgium and Norway training is based on supervised autonomous practice, which is a good model for countries where there is a large proportion of single-handed practices. Even within the UK system there is a lot of variety in how day-release courses work:

- for practice-based trainees only (registrars), or all trainees together
- full day, half day, or block study
- classroom teaching style, or loosely structured on group work lines.

In some places attendance is required and is carefully monitored; in others it is like a drop-in centre for hospital trainees. For reasons that will become apparent later every course is different. The course organizer has a lot of freedom to express the individuality of his approach to education. This is valuable freedom, but it makes it difficult to get to grips with what course organizers do.

There is, however, a consensus that, whatever else they do, their core task is to convene a weekly meeting which trainees (whether practice or hospital based) are entitled to attend. The content and methods of day-release training are explored in detail in Part 2, but for a succinct description it is hard to beat the following statement of aims of the Barts and Holmerton Scheme (Toon et al., 1995):

1 to provide an environment in which continuing peer group support can develop
2 to provide continuing contact with general practice, its clinical orientation and its values, for trainees in the hospital phase
3 to provide learning which can take place only, or most effectively, in groups. This includes role play, problem-solving exercises and the study of the doctor–patient relationship by the Balint method
4 to provide a foundation for self-directed group learning and the avoidance of professional isolation in the doctor's subsequent career.

The job description of the course organizer is considered in Chapter 3.

Exercise 2

1 *Why become a course organizer?*
Many course organizers feel blackmailed or coerced into applying. Whatever your reasons, what do you want to achieve? What do you hope to get out of it?

2 *What are the core activities of the course organizer?*
You cannot begin by doing everything and doing it well. Simplify it to its bare essentials and priorities. (These will vary from place to place.)

I want to be a course organizer because…

I want to achieve…

I expect to gain from being a course organizer in these areas…

The core activities of being a course organizer are…

Exercise 3

You have been appointed to a particular vocational training scheme and to a particular post within the scheme. Who can help you to find out what you are supposed to do?

Exercise 4

In the overall 'family tree' of your region, where do you fit in (see Chapter 15)?

Getting down to business

Like most new course organizers, you will have been a trainer in the same district and participated in the day-release course, so you will have some familiarity with the weekly shape of the course. Previous programmes should be available to you to look over. You may be able to get the outgoing course organizer to provide some guidelines. This will reveal:

1 The structure of the weekly course (Figures 2.1 and 2.2)

Exercise 5

Resources. Is there office space?

Do you have adequate equipment (including a writing board, flip-chart, video, overhead and 35 mm projectors, photocopier, filing cabinet and some storage space)?

Do you have a secretary?

Budget	Who administers this?
	How are speakers paid and who sees to this?
Structure of day-release course	Are other course organizers involved? If so, what is the division of responsibilities?

Curriculum

Is there an established curriculum?

Where can you find out about it?

Who has relevant teaching materials (list of topics, resource people, assessment and test materials, videos etc)?

---

2 The annual cycle of local and regional events such as scheme and regional residentials, special course features and who is responsible for them, fixed dates (term times, project deadlines, exam dates and entry deadlines)
3 Assessment timing, methods and materials.

Visual displays of these are useful, e.g. with a year planner and large filing cards for a synopsis of regular term events, special events which recur, individual major topics and resource persons who are regularly employed (Figure 2.3).

Timetable for half-day release course: template

12.30 pm	Lunchtime meeting – self-resourced by trainees, e.g. journal club
2–3.30 pm	First session (usually structured, didactic)
3.30–3.45 pm	Tea break
3.45–5.15 pm	Second session (usually non-didactic/group based)

Figure 2.1 Sample course structure summary card: half-day timetable.

Generic timetable for day-release course

9.30 am	Coffee, agenda and news
10.15 am	Journal club
11.15 am	Topic I (usually structured/didactic)
12.45 pm	Lunch
2.00 pm	Topic II (usually non-didactic/group based)
3.30 pm	Summarizing, planning

Figure 2.2 Sample course structure summary card: full-day timetable.

First term fixed events: August to December

1 Planning meeting for COs and Directors (early August): content/agenda
2 Initial residential course for trainees (two days, mid-September): content
3 Scheme meetings (full day, rotate around various centres)

- Substance abuse (Derry, October)
- Critical reading (Craigavon, November)
- Minor surgery (Belfast, December)

Note: Summative assessment audit deadline: _____ last entry date for MRCGP: _____

Figure 2.3 Sample course structure summary card: first term.

Course content

A review of former programmes will reveal resource persons and topics which have been used before. Try to find out which were most successful and use them – the ideas may not be fresh but they are a start. Make lists of ideas you like, or priorities with which you can identify, under the headings shown in Figure 2.4.

These are the building blocks of your programme. The 'architecture' – how they are shaped, fitted together and landscaped – is the basis of the course organizer's educational role.

There are two main categories of weekly event – those which are externally resourced and those which are self-resourced (from within the group). There should be a balance of these in any one day's programme.

Topics	Methods	Resources	Other tactics
The consultation	Lecture	Trainers	Journal club
Epidemiology	Discussion with resource person	Other GPs	Videotape
Critical reading	Project	Other health professionals	RCA
Health education	Self-help	Group expert	PCA
Mini-clinics	Workshops	Psychologist (etc)	MEQ
Ischaemic heart disease	Fieldwork (etc)		MCQ (etc)
Anxiety/depression (etc)			

Figure 2.4 Sample course structure summary card: topics and approaches.

You should avoid the temptation to organize the initial programme too tightly. Some blank spaces should be left for discretionary sessions and for taking stock with the trainees or dealing with unfinished business. It is useful and reassuring to have a topic or some resource materials prepared for the unforeseen situation, e.g. when a visiting speaker gets caught in traffic.

The least threatening activities for the course organizer (and the trainees) are clinical lectures with an outside speaker. Frequently this is what new trainees expect. There is a place for these, especially in the early stages; more adventurous ideas can come later.

Even within a set programme of 'safe' clinically oriented material, opportunities arise to:

- get a feeling of how the group functions ('the process')
- explore feelings ('affective learning')
- set exercises ('action learning')
- form opinions about the trainees ('assessment')
- involve them progressively in the curriculum ('active learning').

Such concepts can be explored and developed at a more leisurely pace later.

'Time for me'

When your programme has begun to take shape you should set it aside, relax a bit and turn your attention to longer term planning on such issues as the following.

1 What are your own *learning needs*, e.g. in educational theory and group-work skills?
2 What are the *learning opportunities* available to you: locally (the trainer's workshop, fellow course organizers); regionally (course organizer training meetings); nationally (the ACO training conferences); and personally (appropriate reading)?
3 What *database* do you have: in the library (books, journals, literature search facilities); in the filing system (card index, cabinet files); in your filofax (particulars of resource persons, topics and tactics, resource materials, regional structures, office-bearers); in the course records (notes on trainees, evaluation of sessions, handouts, correspondence, meeting related to the course); and in a daybook (records of each session, decisions made and lessons learned)? Can a computer help?
4 What back-up do you have from your secretary? Enlist her help. She can probably deal with the nuts and bolts of your course better than you can!

As term follows term, you will begin to:

- feel comfortable with an increasing variety of tasks and methods
- take control of the shape and content of the course
- structure your programme less tightly
- give less priority to imparting material and more to building the group self-help
- concentrate on broad themes and the creation of learning opportunities.

Other kinds of task will impinge on your time and ability, for example:

- the trainers' group
- problems and crises of the trainees
- taking part in selection panels for registrars, hospital SHOs, trainers
- taking part in the inspection of training practices
- evaluating or negotiating hospital training posts
- assisting with regional activities such as special educational events for established GPs or trainers
- responding to demands of many unforeseen kinds, some of which may be more related to a GP tutor's function
- learning how to say no.

It is important to keep control of how your role impinges on your other commitments. It is not uncommon for enthusiastic course organizers to fall foul of their partners (medical and marital) through not keeping a balance between competing demands.

Finally, a few slogans:

- have fun, make it fun!
- trainees' ability to learn is not determined by the course organizer's ability
- most course organizers start off feeling inadequate, untrained for the job and apprehensive about their ability
- stop feeling guilty.

Exercise 6

1 Find the Statement of Aims for Vocational Training for your Region. Underline the bits which apply to you
2 Draw up your own 'mission statement' (*see* Figure 2.5)
3 Find out if there is a regional job description for course organizers

---

Summary: Kick-start package for the single-handed new course organizer

1 Identify scheme aims – what are they and who knows them (e.g. the Regional Director)?
2 Find out if there is a job description. Figure 2.6 shows a sample from the West Midlands Region. Focus on the day-release course as your most pressing concern.
3 Find out the course structures from your predecessor or Regional Director. What is the shape of the course each day/term/year? Is it day-release or half-day release?
4 Find out what your resources are – where they are (e.g. district general hospital postgraduate centre) and how they are equipped. Ask your predecessor about useful resource persons and materials, and successful sessions.
5 List likely topics, tactics and methods.
6 Prepare a skeleton programme for the term.
7 Enlist the help of your course secretary for the nuts and bolts of administration.
8 Get on with it (*see* Figure 2.7).
9 Then start thinking about what *you* need, e.g. your learning needs, learning opportunities and your database.
10 Watch your back. Learn to say no.

My course will incorporate the following principles:

- encourage self-help by the trainees
- teach group-work principles (affective learning)
- initiate project work (action/discovery learning)
- use GPs as teachers where possible
- invite specialists as resource persons (and brief them)
- state aims for each session
- evaluate each session
- earmark periodic sessions for SHOs
- plan one term in advance

Figure 2.5 Sample course structure summary card: guidelines.

West Midlands Region VTS Course Organizer Job Description

The role of course organizer is contained in the areas listed below which allow for individual choice and flexibility in the areas s/he wishes to present as representative of her/his work.

The course organizer will:

1 be a principal in general practice
2 have responsibility for organizing learning experience for registrars. The educational principles of these activities should be made explicit. S/he will show an awareness of the special nature of learning in groups
3 have various administrative responsibilities, e.g. liaison with hospital consultants, trainers, regional adviser in general practice etc
4 be responsible for her/his own development as an educationalist
5 be at least in part responsible for the pastoral care of the registrars.

Figure 2.6 Sample of a regional job description for a course organizer (West Midlands) (reproduced with permission).

- Introductions and 'get to know you' exercises
- Invite experienced trainers to brief registrars about priorities for the year
- General outline of GPs' job description and major themes of primary health care
- Guidelines on general reading
- Simple group work discussing problems from the surgery

Figure 2.7 Suggestions for the initial course days.

Scenario: A little education – a dangerous thing?

Best: *Glad to see you, have you started up yet?*

Meeke: *Not yet – next week. By the way, thanks for seeing me so soon after your holiday. I didn't think I would have to call on you just yet, but something has happened and I need your advice.*

Best: *Already! Things move fast when you're a course organizer.*

Meeke: *It's nothing serious, but I met a woman at a party just after I was appointed as CO.*

Best: *Have a drink and spill the beans.*

Meeke: *No, it's not what you're thinking. I barely know her. She's a teacher and she was shocked that I have a teaching job without any training. She talked about the years of education she needed to teach children. I went to the party ready to celebrate and came away feeling like an impostor. Worse than that – inadequate. I feel like backing out of this.*

Best: *Why do you think this is?*

Meeke: *It's not that I'm getting cold feet. I just feel I don't know enough. Sometimes I feel I don't know enough to be a GP, but to teach it as well – to stand up in front of a group of bright young doctors and do anything useful – I don't think I'm ready for that. Maybe in a few years from now...*

Best: *Have you felt like this before?*

Meeke: *Yes, I suppose just after I graduated – the thought of running a hospital ward... then the week before I got married I wanted to run away!*

Best: *So...?*

Meeke: *You think it's stagefright. It's not just that. The day after the party I thought 'I'll do some homework, read up a few books on education and then I'll be ready'. I got a book from the library on the theory and practice of education or some such title. Didn't help a bit – made me worse in fact. I found it woolly, confusing and when I had read a chapter or two I couldn't remember anything I had read – anything useful, that is. I can't get to grips with this education stuff and I don't know how to go about it. It was full of conflicting theories of education. I've tried not to think about it since.*

Best: *This sounds like a reasonably good start. You seem to be taking it seriously – maybe a bit too seriously. You've discovered that there is a lot to learn about being an educator. I have a suggestion – forget the endpoint, start with what you know.*

Meeke: *What I know about education. Not a lot.*

Best: *Think about it – you've been in classrooms, lecture theatres, you've attended seminars and ward rounds, been a GP for years, been a trainer...*

Meeke: *Yes, but...*

Best: *You have a lot of experiences to call on. This may be different but there is a lot of basic common sense you can draw on. How did you manage as a trainer?*

Meeke: *I enjoyed that. We talked about problems. I got the trainee to prepare for tutorials on topics we agreed upon; got out our checklists to see what we hadn't covered; I prepared outline tutorials on a lot of areas and got others in the practice to fill in the bits they could do better; we went over examination papers and put together files of journal articles on broad topics...*

Best: *Stop right there! Any educationalist would translate what you've just said as needs assessment, curriculum planning, formative assessment, experiential and active learning, preparation of educational materials – and you tell me you don't know anything about education!*

Meeke: *Yes, but I don't feel that I know enough about what I'm doing. There are books full of theory and I only know a bit about the practical side. Besides teaching groups is different, isn't it? And some people are born teachers. In the postgraduate centre I don't have the whole training practice as a prop – there's just me and them. How did you start off?*

Best: *I'll tell you in a minute. First, I want to tell you that it doesn't all depend on you. The trainees have their trainers as their first line teacher. You can invite people along to help you out with sessions – just like I invited you a few times to talk to the group – but most important it's not about you teaching them. They're all adults. Your first year with the group might even be your best because you are all learning together – maybe different things, but together. See it as a co-operative venture. There may be some born teachers but if so, they just learn faster how to do it.*

Meeke: *Are you saying that you don't need to know a lot of educational theory to be a course organizer?*

Best: *I suppose I am, but I wouldn't say it too loudly. You asked me how I got started. Much the same as you. My practice was asked to take medical students at a time when general practice was seen simply as a bit of fieldwork for the student. I found that many of them were impressed with the new experience in that they had real things to learn from a GP. I worked around those areas they found different. Vocational training was taking off about that time and we became a training practice. The more I interacted with students and trainees the more I began to value general practice myself. In the early seventies I began to find that there was a growing literature of general practice and education, by GPs for GPs – like the college book, The Future General Practitioner. This introduced me to the education concepts that GPs were finding useful. These days it is a bit like the Bible, well known but not much read. You might have a look at it. The first course organizer in our area involved me in setting up the half-day release course and I really just inherited it when he retired. Becoming a medical teacher of students, a trainer, a course organizer is much more formalized now – but that's because we know what we're about. In the early days we were feeling our way forward. Now our aims and methods have been clarified. You could say that there is now a learning curriculum for GP teachers. Learning by doing is part of our medical culture. Even the educationalists are coming round to seeing the value of that.*

Meeke: *Are you saying that action comes first and theory follows? That's not how medical faculties function – you spend all those years doing basic sciences before you see a patient.*

Best: *Not any more. Whole medical schools have recently been founded on problem-based learning where junior students explore the theory on a need-to-know basis, starting from practice problems.*

Meeke: *A bit of James Bond there – the need to know. So what do I need to know before I start?*

Best: *Your question reminds me of a cartoon I saw once – an old grey-beard in a bath chair, the wall covered in medical diplomas and the caption 'By the time he was fully qualified he was too old to do anything'. Maybe life is too short for reading all the texts on education that you might need, even if you wanted to.*

Meeke: *Surely you're not saying it doesn't matter?*

Best: *Not at all. First, what you need to know is yourself – what you want to achieve, how committed you are to being a teacher. You know a lot about general practice and how to relate to patients in a way that respects their dignity and autonomy, facilitating them in identifying their problems and needs, and motivating them to work on them. There you have the basic approach to education – how not to make a situation worse. Educationalists call it 'the principle of adult learning'. You can read books on that later; then they will make some sense to you.*

Meeke: *But is this not putting the cart before the horse – the practice before the theory? Worse – it's almost as if the two are not connected at all and that good practice can exist without the theory.*

Best: *Yes, perhaps. Horses and carts are different – after all, they come out of different stables (in a manner of speaking) but they are linked to one another. The reality is in what they are meant to do. Overload either and you create problems. As the horse gets used to the cart they become a more efficient unit. But enough of folk wisdom, what are you learning about your real question?*

Meeke: *I'm still struggling with the idea that you don't have to know much about teaching to be a teacher. But I feel better about it. I have been anxious because I think there are dangers involved in teaching – both to the trainees and me. They say a little knowledge is a dangerous thing. I've been warned about that by the lady at the party, so I'll go carefully, start simple and feel my way and do a bit of reading as I go along, find out what all the jargon in the books is about. It's very off-putting – the jargon, I mean.*

Best: *What is jargon to one person is the technical terms of another's discipline. For example, you have just described reflection in action – you'll come across that one again. A lot of experienced trainers and course organizers are doing diplomas in medical education now to make sense of what they have been doing all along and develop their skills so they can do it better. What they discover is that there is no such thing as educational theory. There are a lot of theories of education, many of them conflicting. That doesn't mean they are wrong but fashions change as one after another gains ascendance. Hence all the jargon.*

Meeke: *So what's the point of all of this educational stuff if it doesn't come to any conclusions?*

Best: *A lot of fields of knowledge are inconclusive. That doesn't make them worthless – quite the contrary, it makes you think about what you are doing and why, and how to embrace change rather than settling for rigid rules. Education is about processes and models and guidelines rather than learning the right way.*

Meeke: *So, for now, I just get on with it and use what I know. That sounds like a common sense approach. I think I need a few props, things to get me going, like:*

- *an outline timetable*
- *a list of straightforward topics and activities*
- *a list of local people I can ask to conduct sessions… and some more sessions like this as I go along.*

Best: *Enough to be going on with. As for educationalism, let me show you a few notes I took down from a book I read recently, if I can find the right card in my index.*

- If education is strong on common sense it is also weak on theory to the point where people question its credentials as a discipline or field
- In reality there is very little educational theory, although there is a great deal of other kinds of theory in education
- In general, the problem of educational theory is not that there is too much, but that there is too little
- Education as a field has largely failed to develop its own characteristic models, framework or concept and remains a largely derivative discipline
- Is systematic training in educational theory possible? If there is no (central) theory or model, how can we establish a connection between what the teacher teaches and what the learner learns – between input and output?
- There are two main branches of educational theory – what is taught (curriculum) and how (pedagogy, androgogy)

Figure 2.8 Dr Best's file card: taken from Squires, 1994.

Exercise 7

Rank the following paradigms ranging from that which you agree with most – 1 – to that which you agree with least – 6. 'Paradigm' here means a general approach to or way of thinking about something, and might cover several theories or models of the same type. You may want to add another paradigm of your own if you think that none represents it adequately.

1 **Common sense**

Teaching/training is a common sense activity because everyone has been exposed to it for many years and because it shares many of the features of normal human communication and interaction. We learn to teach/train by drawing on our experience and informal knowledge of the activity, and using our common sense to develop that. Formal training is therefore unnecessary.

Exercise 7 continued

2 Art

Some people have a natural gift or talent for teaching/training which can be developed but not created in the first place. Teachers/trainers are essentially born not made – much depends on personality and style – and the process remains instinctive and mysterious in many ways. We learn to teach by refining our instincts and judgements; and initial selection is more important than training. Indeed, training may be impossible.

3 Craft

Teaching/training is largely a matter of methods, skills, techniques and procedures. Like all crafts, it is learned primarily through on-the-job apprenticeship, observation, imitation, practice and feedback under the gradually decreasing supervision of an expert practitioner. It is a clearly transparent activity which almost anyone can carry out with the proper training.

4 Rational activity

Teaching/training is a rational, systematic process and like all such processes involves identifying aims and objectives, choosing and implementing appropriate strategies to fulfil them and evaluating the outcomes. We learn to teach/train essentially by learning to analyse, design, deliver and evaluate within a broad 'systems' framework.

5 Applied science

Like other professions, teaching/training is based on certain underlying theories, laws or principles which in this case relate to the process of learning and development. Without such principles, teaching/training degenerates into a matter of habit, trial and error, individual intuition or cultural relativism. We learn to teach/train by understanding such underlying principles and putting them into practice.

6 Reflective practice

Teaching/training is essentially a practical rather than a theoretical activity and involves many complex, specific and often implicit rules-of-thumb and judgements which are grounded in practice and developed through experience. We learn to teach by reflecting on, drawing out and articulating these to ourselves and others, and using them to inform and influence our practice.

(Reproduced with permission from Squires, 1994)

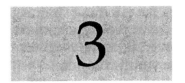

3

What is a course organizer?

Introduction

The need for course organizers is obvious only in retrospect. Most other developed countries do not have a real equivalent, nor do the major hospital specialty training schemes in the UK. The innovative nature of the post is not diminished by the observation that it was conceived in haste and born in compromise. Course organizers emerged at a time of innovation in general practice, following the establishment of the College of General Practitioners (in 1952), the GP Charter (in 1965), the appearance of the first university departments of general practice, and the appointment in 1972 of the first regional advisers. According to Pereira Gray (1986), the introduction of course organizers was so rapid that there was no time to plan or negotiate their job description or remuneration. In effect the course organizer was defined as a trainer with a group instead of a trainee, and his job was to act as a link between the trainees and the Regional Adviser (Director.) It was envisaged that he could respond to trainees' enquiries, plan release courses, negotiate hospital posts, liaise with trainer workshops, participate in trainer approval visits and give briefings to the regional advisers.

The course organizer's role has developed rapidly since then. Course organizers now have their own association (the Association of Course Organizers (ACO)) which runs educational courses and conferences, and a journal dealing with vocational training issues (*see* Chapter 15). In 1992, the level of remuneration was upgraded from the trainer's grant to the second point on the NHS consultant scale.

Course organizers have been described by the Royal College of General Practitioners as one of the major successes in vocational training (RCGP, 1989). Our social work colleagues frequently complain that they are being handicapped by the proliferation of statutory functions. Course organizers, on the other hand, suffer from a lack of such official guidelines. For GP registrars the trainer is the key educator. The course

	EDUCATIONAL	MANAGERIAL	PROFESSIONAL
	MOTIVATION		
ESSENTIAL	Teaching ability Group leader Inspirational	Organizer Accessible Negotiator	Good GP Approachable Up to date
	COMMUNICATOR		
	SENSITIVE AND SELF-AWARE		
DESIRABLE	Attended course for organizers Lateral thinker Counsellor Breadth of vision Trainer	Delegator	MRCGP Innovator Counsellor
	CHARISMATIC		
CONTRA- INDICATIONS	Inflexible	Over-committed	Intolerant partners Burnt out

Figure 3.1 Criteria for course organizers (Styles, 1986).

2 for those who work in teams, some rational division of labour should be agreed even though each individual should be capable of 'covering' for his team colleague(s).

The quality attributes of the course organizer shown in Figure 3.1 were compiled by a working party during the second ACO national conference (Styles, 1986). Beliefs and values appropriate to course organizers are further explored in Chapter 4.

The only definitive recent contribution to the evolving scene came from the Annual General Meeting of the ACO in 1995 which adopted the job description shown in Figure 3.2. It reflects the changing culture within the NHS by recognizing the distinction between core functions which represent the national consensus, and optional functions which apply to individual circumstances. These may form a basis for local negotiation and separate remuneration. The inclusion of 'budget-holding' as a core function is not universally accepted.

GP VOCATIONAL TRAINING COURSE ORGANIZER JOB DESCRIPTION

The vocational training course organizer is a GP medical postgraduate teacher and educational manager, working within the framework of the Regional Adviser in General Practice and the Postgraduate Dean.

BASIC REQUIREMENTS
- Fully registered medical practitioner
- Satisfactory completion of preliminary training course
- Principal in contract with the FHSA, current or recent

ACCOUNTABILITY
- To the Regional Adviser for General Practice

APPOINTMENT
- Sessional, by agreement with Regional Adviser
- Payment on 2nd point of Consultant scale (currently)
- Superannuable post

The principal task of the course organizer is to support the professional development of GP registrars and SHOs on Schemes, encouraging autonomy in the learners, and to develop their sensitivity to patients' needs, using group learning approaches in particular.

The job description for course organizers will include the following core functions. Some course organizers may also include some optional functions as part of their job. These will be locally negotiated and resourced.

FUNCTIONS
CORE
- *Educational*
  - Recruitment, interviewing and appointment of GP registrars and SHOs
  - Development, planning and provision of training programme for GP registrars and SHOs on Schemes
  - Monitoring training programme
  - Formative assessment with GP registrars and SHOs on Schemes
  - Continuing programme of personal professional development
  - Educational liaison with other course organizers regionally and nationally

- *Management*
  - Business planning
  - Budget holding
  - Resource management
  - Production of annual reports
  - Liaison with GP and hospital trainers

- *Pastoral*
  - Support and advice for GP registrars and SHOs on Schemes
  - Support and advice for trainers, hospital consultants and other course organizers

OPTIONAL (locally determined)
- Non-parochial use of skills in summative assessment of GP registrars
- Training appointment and monitoring of trainers
- Representation on regional and national educational committees
- Development and use of specific educational skills
- Remedial work with poorly achieving and non-competent GP registrars
- Careers advice to junior doctors

Figure 3.2 ACO job description of the course organizer, 1995.

Who is the course organizer?

Approximately 1% of GPs are course organizers. In 1985, only 4% of course organizers were women and 2% were in single-handed practice, which may be a reflection on the demanding workload and diversity of the job. The typical profile of the course organizer suggests that he:

- is male in his forties
- is from a large group training practice
- is a former trainer who has spent 10–15 years in practice as a principal
- is a member of the RCGP
- has spent less than five years in course organizing.

There is no evidence or reason to believe that this profile has changed substantially since 1985.

The search for a definition

A course organizer's functions are in some ways as diverse as those of a GP. Various aspects of the job heighten this impression.

- Both are open-ended commitments whose contractual features bear little relationship to the actual job.
- Trying to define the curriculum is like trying to define health care – it is difficult to discern the boundaries.
- The course organizer's wider responsibilities are related to the undefined needs of a defined population.

One of the most successful and enduring definitions of the GP is the Leeuwenhorst statement. This provides a useful template for developing the following definition of a course organizer.

The course organizer as the generalist of vocational training

- The course organizer is a GP who has a part-time contract of responsibility for the education of a group of trainees.
- His responsibilities relate mostly to the day-release course, but he will liaise with those providing training in hospitals (consultants) and in approved practices (trainers).
- His aim is to oversee the educational needs of the group and identify the problems of specific trainees at an early stage to that corrective action can be taken (formative assessment).

- He will integrate knowledge, skills and attitudes in his formulation of educational tasks.
- He will respond with pastoral concern to any problem raised by the trainees as individuals or as a group.
- He will facilitate the trainees towards self-learning, audit and continuing medical education.
- The time span of vocational training means that he can keep an eye on the progress of the individual trainees and the group, and build up a relationship of trust.
- He will enlist the help of trainers, other GP teachers, consultants and resource persons (medical and non-medical) to provide learning opportunities.
- He will liaise with the Regional Director, trainers' workshop and hospital consultants about the organization and content of vocational training.
- He will be conversant with enough educational theory and practice to be able to function in direct teaching, curriculum planning, assessment and administration to promote the professional and personal growth of the trainees.
- He will recognize that he also has other responsibilities in relation to general practice and the wider profession.

A course organizer is not:

- omniscient and omnicompetent
- a trainer (he has group concerns which go beyond those of the individuals involved)
- a teacher (he is more like a conductor of an orchestra: he does not have to be able to play all the instruments himself)
- Sisyphus (pushing the same stone up the same hill year after year).

Future trends

The historical trend from 1970 has been one of incremental change. There was gradual convergence of early regional experiments to form a recognizable job profile which allows for considerable local variation but is firmly rooted in clinical and educational practice. The extensive changes in general practice since the 1990 contract, the influence of locality and practice-based commissioning and the purchaser–provider split have changed the culture of primary health care. Inevitably this will be reflected in how education for general practice is delivered. This could take a variety of forms.

The course organizer could develop along the lines of either provider, as at present, or purchaser of vocational training at local level (Percy and Pitts, 1994). Any introduction of budget-holding as a core activity for course organizers would pave the way for a greater emphasis on the purchaser role, with devolution of the training budget from regional to local level. In recent years a drop in recruitment to general practice training has forced Regional Directors to examine the need for manpower planning. It would be in their interest to devise a contractual system whereby, through a block grant, each vocational training scheme produced a defined number of fully trained doctors, congruent with local need. Recent national policy is introducing a longer period of practice-based training (at least 18 months), with probable reduction in the hospital requirement (Calman, 1995). This may further shift the emphasis of training provision in the direction of locally sensitive need.

The Association of Course Organizers adopted a policy that the full three year period of training should be based on general practice (ACO, 1997). This implies rotation round a sequence of complementary practice-related placements. Training practices would then be the primary providers of training, with other providers (such as individual hospital departments) being commissioned as required. This will result in complex funding arrangements with a strong local emphasis. Course organizers would have an essential role in co-ordinating and monitoring such developments.

Within this scenario the day-release course would have a high profile. All trainees on a local scheme could be expected to attend consistently over the full period of training. It would, therefore, provide the only thread of continuity through the training pathway. Provision would have to be made for trainees to transfer between schemes without loss of momentum. This would require a system for accrediting the unique training pathway of each individual, with the use of portfolio-based learning and a credit accumulation transfer system (CATS) within a national, perhaps European, framework.

It is possible to envisage the course organizer as a local co-ordinator of education:

- administering a block grant, purchasing educational services from local trainers and other providers
- leading an educational consortium representing the educational skill-mix available locally
- co-ordinating an integrated, three year day-release course based on the skill-mix of the consortium
- managing the accreditation process for all local trainees.

Membership of a consortium could be widely defined to include local medical and non-medical educators. Its remit might be expanded to encompass the continuing education needs of the locality including multi-disciplinary education and training programmes with other professions allied to medicine (PAMs).

This is a nightmare scenario for course organizers who enjoy being teachers. It would be a great loss if we were deprived of our central source of job satisfaction and distinctive identity by the necessity to adopt an increasingly managerial role. However, many GPs have successfully assimilated parallel changes through the fundholding scheme without ceasing to be GPs. Much of the administrative load could be devolved to appropriately skilled non-medical personnel. This may not be the 'other side of the moon' scenario, but the first crescent of the hunter's moon beginning to appear.

Scenario: A dialogue

Meeke: *We've had three sessions of the day-release course so far, and it's chaos! On paper I have 20 trainees. Half of them are still in SHO posts in five different hospitals, most of them haven't put in an appearance yet. As for the trainees in GP posts, some of them are just out of their houseman year doing a sandwich scheme, some are half-way through their practice year after joining and out of sync with the rest who have all done the usual rotations. One is on maternity leave, two more are on honeymoon. One has a PhD and another is older than I am. I don't see when I am going to get them all together and, if I do, whether anything I teach will mean anything to all of them since they all seem to be different.*

Best: *You've obviously had a fairly effective 'get to know you' session with the group. That's a good start and it's where group work begins. You've also discovered the important basic points of adult education: first, each adult learner is an individual with a unique set of experiences, expectations and learning styles. They all come from different work situations and have different pressures. All these things complicate your task as an educator. Ask any Open University or extramural teacher – they'll know what you're talking about. Can you see what the positive values of that are?*

Meeke: *I suppose they're likely to have different approaches to a problem, see things differently and maybe disagree more than I'd expected. They might learn a lot from each other if I get them going.*

Best: *Exactly – group interaction. That's what makes teaching adults exciting.*

Meeke: *But it's so unpredictable. I'd rather just get on with teaching as that's what I enjoyed as a trainer and what I became a course organizer for.*

Best: *Remember, for every individual learning style there is a corresponding teaching style. You'll soon learn how to mix input with discovery, task with process work, affective learning with action learning, how to modulate a group exercise without them noticing it, so that the talkers listen and the quiet ones discover they can express themselves. You'll find…*

Meeke: *Hey, hang on, that's all jargon!*

Best: *Sorry, but what you call jargon, I prefer to call technical terms.*

Meeke: *Okay. Can you just translate it into doctor-speak?*

Best: *With pleasure. Would you accept that general practice is becoming patient centred? And that trainers in teaching practices are being encouraged to be trainee centred, to match the training activities to the individual trainee's needs? In much the same way the course organizer, who is the trainer to the trainee group, must be group centred. You can treat the group as you would a patient – respecting its autonomy, diagnosing its needs and disorders, intervening preventively, treating any malfunction and referring (when necessary) to other experts if you are out of your depth. But it helps to know something about the processes, skills and resources involved. Hence the jargon. And just as the patient's health is his own, the trainees must be helped*

> to become responsible for their own learning process. You are a resource to them just like the GP is the front-line resource to his patients.

Meeke: I think I'll enjoy doing all that, but I don't like assessment. Isn't it a bit authoritarian?

Best: It's just a way of saying what you're doing and whether it's delivering the goods. There is nothing new about it. Look back to educational texts written 30 years ago. It's there in the education cycle under different names.

Meeke: Maybe I'll start with the educational stuff and leave the groupie stuff for a while. I can imagine how some of that lot will react when I suggest they sit around and hold hands and talk to each other about their feelings!

Part 2

The educational role of
the course organizer

Overview

Course organizing is primarily an educational task. There is much common ground with teachers in all health care disciplines.

In the school system, teacher training is becomingly increasingly based on supervised practice in the classroom. Many new course organizers do not have the benefit of an experienced mentor who can regularly supervise their work in the day-release course. This means that you may have to undertake a good deal of action learning for yourself. Your previous experience as a GP and trainer will be of great value initially.

Education is a very practical discipline. Nevertheless, successful education requires a grasp of the theoretical issues which give cohesion and direction to the activities involved in becoming as good a teacher as possible.

This Part outlines the aspects of education that a course organizer needs to know about, and provides summaries of the main theoretical issues. The practical implications of these will be considered.

When you have been in the job for a while, the relevance of the theory will become more apparent. As you identify educational areas which you wish to explore in more detail, you can look out for short courses and further reading to meet your particular needs.

Chapter 4 begins with the *context* of vocational training and stresses the need for an *educational philosophy*, the value system which guides your priorities. These, together with two major concepts – the needs of *adult learners* and their *learning styles* – lay the foundation for the rest of Part 2 which consists of five interlocking units: Chapter 5, on *educational methods*, discusses the skills, activities and resources you are likely to employ. Chapter 6 deals with the *assessment* of trainees, while Chapter 7 discusses the place of *examinations* in vocational training and how the main ones are structured. Finally Chapter 8, on *curriculum development*, gives some guidelines for preparing the teaching programme and Chapter 9 carries this through to preparation for continuing learning.

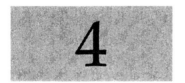

4

The course organizer
as educator

Introduction

The course organizer is first and foremost a GP, and therefore has to acquire educational expertise somehow without the luxury of an extended period of supervised teacher training on the job or substantial study leave from the surgery.

Our survey of the early needs of course organizers (Part 1) shows that most feel unprepared for this role. They would welcome some rigorous preparation, a personal tutor and a practical textbook. However, in practice, they often inherit the job and begin by getting on with what their predecessor has set up, relying on their previous experience. Their role as health educators for their patients gives GPs opportunities to discover skills which are common to all educational settings. Many also have experience of one-to-one teaching, as trainers. Pragmatism is a great teacher. You can put your experience to work right away, perhaps with the help and guidance of an experienced colleague or predecessor (like Dr Best in the scenarios) and supplement this with reading and attending short courses.

There is nothing to apologize for in this approach. The medical tradition has always asserted that its teachers should be active practitioners who reflect on what they are doing and communicate their experience using the apprenticeship model and 'simple' educational techniques including lectures, laboratory practicals and bedside case discussion. As teachers they have been part-time amateurs, more concerned with the message than the medium. This has stood the test of time because of the institutionally based history of medical training.

Vocational training for general practice is rooted in this tradition. More recently modification has become necessary to take account of the patient-centred and community-based medicine of primary care. This creates educational challenges which are relatively new, because the discipline of general practice is still finding a methodology which is distinct from that of hospital practice.

These educational challenges include:

- encompassing the huge and expanding field of clinical general practice (together with the community perspectives of health promotion, administration, management, audit and research)
- developing the prospective GP's interpersonal skills to maximize 'the exceptional potential of the consultation in general practice' (Stott, 1979)
- equipping them with autonomous learning skills
- preparing them for a way of life which allows them to integrate their work, their own well-being and that of their families.

The course organizer's role has become that of an educational overseer, managing the transition from one educational tradition to another. The practice trainees are at a transitional state in more than one sense. Professionally, they are stepping from institution to community. Educationally, they are moving from the 'high-tech', disease-centred setting to a relatively 'low-tech', patient-centred approach to delivery of health care. Socially, they are losing their hospital peer-group which has been their work setting since student days. Personally, many are beginning to experience the demands of real life: marriage, mortgage and parenthood. In short, they are becoming *adult learners*.

This phase of multiple transition constitutes a crisis in the technical sense. They have new learning needs in every area of life. It would be regrettable if this were not matched with a correspondingly wide array of learning opportunities.

This is the educational setting of the course organizer. To do it justice, you need to develop an educational strategy which is comprehensive and realistic. There are six main components.

1 *Educational philosophy*: your 'mission statement' of values and beliefs.
2 *Educational framework*: the areas of educational theory which are essential to the role, in particular the needs of adult learners and their learning styles.
3 *Educational methods*: the skills, activities and resources at your disposal.
4 *Educational assessment* of your efforts, what is happening and how it might be improved.
5 *Examinations*: their place in assessment and accreditation for professional life.
6 *Curriculum development*: the considerations which govern the priorities in putting together and running an educational programme for trainees.

The rest of this chapter looks at the first two components in some detail.

Educational philosophy

This is the formulation of the beliefs and values which underlie the educational process. It is concerned with the ethics and attitudes of the educator, the aims, contents and priorities of the programme, and the educational vision which forms the basis of the learning contract between the educator and the learners. It should:

- foster vision and aspiration, and not be constrained by practicalities
- clarify, rather than obscure, the day-to-day aspects of the job
- bring to light the assumptions which underlie what we do
- identify priorities and methods
- take account of the problems of defining goals and assessing progress towards them
- be subjected to evaluation through reflection and dialogue with the learners and other educators
- develop with the individual course organizer's growth as an educator.

If we do not have an educational philosophy there is a danger that:

- education will become training and training will become indoctrination
- the individuality, creativity and dignity of the learners will be suppressed
- the integrity and enthusiasm of the educator will diminish
- the possibilities for change and growth will be extinguished.

Our current terminology is unhelpful in developing a philosophy. Consider the *values* implicit in the following terms: trainer, trainee, course organizer, vocational, training and day-release. There are implications of a hierarchy, a mechanistic learning process, the compartmentalization of learning and working, and a defined endpoint achievable by a course of training. There is nothing wrong with these terms so long as we are not constrained by them and they are seen merely as shorthand for a more flexible, comprehensive and profound analysis.

These issues affect you as a course organizer, more than any other medical teacher, because your role is unique and ill defined, and because you are not the primary educator in the system as its exists. This is based on the apprenticeship model with the focus on the one-to-one learning relationship between the trainee and the practice trainer or hospital consultant teacher. The course organizer's distinctive place is as an overseer of the complete process (Hayden, 1996). You are a resource person to the trainee group without the inherent power of an employer or a judge of competence who can give or withhold the necessary certificates. Paradoxically, this lack of responsibility may be among your greatest strengths, because it:

- permits the blurring of the teacher–learner axis
- allows openness in sharing views, problems and vulnerabilities (affective learning)
- shifts the focus of attention to the group rather than the teacher as the resource for learning (peer learning)

- validates the worth of 'soft' knowledge (the learning of higher order abilities) without detracting from the value of 'hard' facts
- allows for divergent thinking and interdisciplinary learning – the cross-linkages which bridge the gap between knowledge and competence.

From these perspectives it is possible to formulate a code of practice. Two examples are offered here. One is in the form of the personal manifesto of a course organizer. The other is the statement of educational philosophy of the ACO (McEvoy, 1992).

Example: Educational manifesto of a course organizer

1 Time on the day-release course is at a premium: it will be regarded as quality time.
2 The day-release course will supplement, not duplicate, the function of the hospital training posts and the training practice.
3 The educational activities of the day-release course will be primarily trainee centred.
4 The values, dignity and individuality of each trainee will be respected in all day-release course activities.
5 Group work and peer learning will be emphasized as educational strategies.
6 The curriculum of the day-release course will emphasize transferable skills and knowledge; the development of methodology, principles, strategies and values; it will seek to move from the particular to the general.
7 Teaching methods will be selectively used to maximize the involvement of the learner; resource persons will be selectively employed and carefully briefed in such a way that active learning is promoted.
8 Participants will be encouraged to identify their own learning needs and enlist help in meeting them.
9 The personal and professional well-being of all members of the course will be included in the overt curriculum and will be among the educational and pastoral concerns of the course organizer.
10 Formal and informal assessment procedures will be employed to evaluate the effectiveness of the course and the progress of the learners.

Example 2: Statement of core educational beliefs of the Association of Course Organizers

1 The course organizer is a medical teacher whose educational skills enable him or her to recognize and provide learning opportunities for trainees, and perhaps other learners, in a variety of settings. Course organizers have special skills in small group teaching.

2 The course organizer is particularly concerned with fostering the autonomy of the learner.

3 The course organizer aims to facilitate the learner's professional development and personal growth in areas such as reflectiveness, integrity, ethical awareness and sensitivity to the needs of patients.

4 The trainee-centred emphasis of the course organizer reflects the patient-centred nature of general practice.

5 Course organizers have a special concern for formative assessment while being effective in supporting learners as they prepare for appropriate summative assessment.

6 The Association of Course Organizers aims to provide educational support in the application and development of these priorities.

Educational framework of course organizing

For our purposes as course organizers, educational theory can be reduced to two main themes: adult learning (who are the learners and what do they need?) and cognitive style (how do they learn?).

Adult learners

Brookfield (1986) identified six main characteristics of adult learners.

1 They are not beginners, but are in a continuing process of growth.
2 They bring with them a package of experiences and values, each one unique.
3 They come to education with intentions.
4 They bring expectations about the learning process.
5 They have competing interests – the realities of their lives.
6 They already have their own set patterns of learning.

Adult education is therefore most productive when:

• a climate conducive to learning is established
• learning activities seem to have some relevance to the learners' circumstances
• the learner's past experiences are used in the learning process
• the learners are engaged in the design of learning
• learners are encouraged to be self-directed
• the educator functions as a facilitator rather than as a didactic instructor
• individual learners' needs and learning styles are taken into account.

Rogers (1988) wrote: '*The purpose of adult education is to help them to learn, not to teach them all they know and thus stop them from carrying on learning.*' Schön (1983) stressed the distinction between pedagogy (the teaching of children) and androgogy (adult learning).

Pedagogy is akin to training. It encourages convergent thinking and rote learning. It is compulsory, centred on the teacher and the imparting of information with minimal control by the learner. This is reminiscent of the process of medical teaching up to the level of vocational training.

Androgogy, by contrast, is about education as freedom. It encourages divergent thinking and active learning. Whatever the curriculum content, there is certainty about the outcomes. Learning and teaching roles are blurred. It emphasizes the assimilation of learning with life experience and peer learning. It is voluntary, learner oriented and opens up vistas for continued learning. Adults need to feel independent and in control of their learning. Trainees appear to be in a transitional state from pedagogy to androgogy and from course-oriented working patterns to self-directed continued learning. Mismanagement of the transition can inhibit the emergence of suitable continuing learning patterns, with long-term consequences for the new GP's career. However, attempts to make the trainees responsible for their own curriculum and learning needs often result in silence and resentment. This polarization is unnecessary. Perhaps 'learner sensitive' is a better term than 'learner centred'.

Exercise 8
My educational philosophy is based on the following principles...

Exercise 9
Topics for day-release course will be chosen by the following criteria...

Resource persons for the day-release course will be chosen according to the following guidelines...

Cognitive style

The literature of vocational training, and education in general, makes frequent reference to cognitive or learning style, but it is difficult to find a succinct definition. Riding and Cheema (1991) carried out a literature review which identified over 30 attributes related to many different models of cognitive style. They conclude that there is no single underlying concept. Much of the literature on cognitive style is reminiscent of the magazine horoscope, or well-meaning efforts to explain away the reality of the range of ability, i.e. IQ.

Psychologists assure us that this is not the case, but that there is a variety of personal abilities which are not all measurable by the same psychometric tool. The Scottish Council for Postgraduate Medical Education (SCPME, 1991) gave perhaps the simplest formulation of this: *'Everyone learns in different ways so it is important to find out what works well for you'*.

Most people agree, however, on a few central concepts.

1 *Cognitive style* is a person's typical or habitual mode of problem solving, thinking, perceiving or remembering.
2 *Learning style* is cognitive style in action in the learning situation. The two are frequently used interchangeably. Learning styles are not IQ dependent.
3 *Teaching style* is the mirror image of learning style, i.e. the strategies followed by the teacher, either intrinsically or as a deliberate response to the needs of the learners.
4 *Learning strategies* are the ways adopted to cope with learning tasks and problems. Where learning style constitutes a problem, learning strategies may be elaborated to compensate. Unlike styles which are relatively fixed for the individual, strategies may vary and be learned and developed.
5 *Instructional preference* is the individual's choice of environment in which to learn, e.g. in group discussion, by action learning, by dialogue, by video/audio/interactive disk or alone in the library. This suggests a spectrum of preference from social to autonomous learning.

Individuals may function in more than one style, employing them in different situations. Some individuals may show excessive reliance on one style, exhibiting a 'learning pathology' which may need special help. The teacher who is aware that his own cognitive style influences his teaching style should also try to diversify.

There is no need to feel inadequate in the presence of colleagues who can quote chapter and verse on a given topic when you can only summarize the current literature. You just have different cognitive styles.

The type of assessment used has been shown to influence the learner's approach to learning (Newble and Entwhistle, 1986). Objective testing methods such as multiple choice questionnaires and endpoint assessment do not suit everyone. To be valid there should be a variety of assessment approaches, applied at various times and with an emphasis on formative assessment (*see* Chapter 5) accompanied by 'remedial teaching' when, for example, a trainee appears to present a problem of behaviour or performance. Such remedial teaching may take the form of identifying the trainee's learning style in order to work with or diversify it.

The need for adaptability on both sides was neatly expressed over a century ago by Leo Tolstoy, in his essay 'On teaching the rudiments': *'Every teacher must...by regarding every imperfection in the pupil's comprehension, not as a defect in the pupil, but as a defect of his own instruction, endeavour to develop in himself the ability of discovering new methods.'*

It is easy to get bogged down in a mass of empirical studies. A synopsis of current models will give an idea of what people mean when they talk about learning styles. The extensive review article by Riding and Cheema (1991) covers the ground in great detail.

Learning process model

Honey and Mumford (1986) postulated a four-stage process of learning and equated each with a type of person who responds selectively to that stage. Neighbour (1990) summarized these as follows:

1 welcome new ideas and experiences – Activists
2 reflection; implications considered and data gathered – Reflectors
3 assimilation; new material is integrated, incorporated with experience and improved – Theorists
4 trying out new knowledge – Pragmatists.

Honey and Mumford's learning style questionnaire is instructive and fun to do, although the categories are probably not mutually exclusive.

Personality model

The Myers–Briggs Type Indicator classifies personality traits into four bipolar scales (Myers, 1962):

- feeling – thinking
- sensing – intuitive
- introverted – extroverted
- perceiving – judging.

The permutations of these produce a matrix of 16 categories. The individual's place in the matrix can be correlated with guidelines concerning vocational direction and learning needs. It has been standardized on populations of US medical students and doctors.

Approach-based model (Newble and Entwhistle, 1986)

Derived from studies on college students in the USA, this model suggests three distinct approaches to learning.

1 Deep. Such students are either *serialist*, employing the step-by-step approach favoured by science students, or *holistic* (like typical arts students, discerning themes and variations), or *versatile* (employing both methods – these are the most

academically successful). This style is fostered by the problem-based learning approach (Newble and Clarke, 1986) (*see* Chapter 8).

2 Superficial. Such students memorize facts and examples, either actively (with motivation they may succeed), or passively (without interest, and resultant success).

3 Strategic. Such students may make the grade by 'playing the system'.

Curry's onion model

In this somewhat 'aromatic' model it is suggested that all teaching/learning measures can be grouped into three strata like the skins of an onion (Curry, 1983).

1 The outer layer is the instructional preference (environmental factors which are easily perceived and easily influenced).

2 The middle layer is the information processing style, which can be modified by learning strategies. Learning style inventories measure this.

3 The core is the cognitive personality style – the approach used to adapt and assimilate information. The Myers–Briggs questionnaire measures this.

Riding and Cheema's model

This asserts that there are only two truly independent groups of learning style attributes.

1 The verbalizer–imager axis. This correlates with Eysenck's Introvert–Extrovert scale. Verbalizers tend to be extroverts who perform well on verbal tests and learn best from texts; visualizers tend to be introverts who find concrete, visual material easier to comprehend and recall.

2 The holistic–analytic axis. Correlates include a large cluster of bipolar attributes.

Holistic type
- Field dependence
- Impulsive style
- Leveller (wanting to simplify things)
- Divergent thinking
- Holistic (with global concepts)

Analytic type
- Field independence
- Reflective
- Sharpener (perceiving complexity)
- Convergent thinking
- Serialist (with linear concepts)

The most significant of these is the concept of field dependence/independence which may be summarized as follows:

Field-dependent type
- Relates to external frame of reference
- Requires much interaction with peers and teachers

Field-independent type
- Internal frame of reference
- Requires little interaction with peers and teachers

- Functions well in groups
- Responds to external reinforcement
- Needs structured work
- Good interpersonal skills, socially perceptive
- Needs help with problem solving

- Functions as an individual, has self-defined goals
- Intrinsic reinforcement
- Structures own learning needs
- Needs help in developing social, co-operative learning skills and empathy
- Good at problem solving

Field-dependent teachers:

- prefer interaction with learners, involving them in the content of teaching and encouraging them to formulate principles themselves
- are reluctant to express critical feedback
- are concerned with positive attitudes and classroom atmosphere.

By contrast, field-independent teachers:

- prefer formal approaches
- emphasize their own standards
- formulate and encourage the application of principles
- correct what they see as errors
- focus on subject content and are relatively uninterested in ambience and attitudes.

Guidelines

This theory can be translated into practical guidelines.

1 Recognize that your own learning style(s) will strongly influence your teaching style.
2 Be prepared to study and practise teaching methods which are not central to your 'comfort zone'.
3 Recognize that trainees, as adult learners, will come with a variety of fixed concepts about learning.
4 Modes of assessment should be realistic and varied. In assessing your own efforts as a course organizer you should not expect the trainees to be unanimous in their feedback.
5 Avoid relating particular learning styles to intelligence. We probably select our good trainees in much the same way as patients identify a 'good' GP. It may be equally difficult to define the grounds for such selection.

Guidelines for 'remedial teaching'

1 Provide a variety of teaching methods to recruit the best efforts of the various styles. Methods can be both formal and interactive, and involve personal study and group work. They may include discussions and projects and the use of verbal and visual media. Emphasis should be on both concept and evidence.
2 Accept the idiosyncratic trainee, but think about setting tasks which require structured performance. Perhaps he is a divergent thinker with more to offer to peer learning than the conforming problem-solver.
3 If you identify strongly 'field-dependent' trainees, respond with structured work, specific goals and encouragement. Field-independent trainees may benefit from involvement in co-operative group activities and interprofessional learning, although they may resist this.
4 As course organizer you cannot meet the exacting requirements required of all types at all times but you can enhance growth possibilities through peer learning by facilitating experience of, and exposure to, individuals in the group who have differing styles.

Exercise 10

Can you identify your own preferred learning style?
How does it correlate with your preferred methods of teaching?
Think of a trainee who has a markedly different style from yours.
What can you do to really meet his needs?

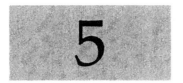

Educational methods

Introduction

There is a bewildering variety of educational methods and teaching techniques available. The list of methods in this chapter can be regarded as a formulary of drugs, each with its individual profile of purpose, side-effects and interactions (and perhaps its own toxic, allergenic and idiosyncratic properties, LD50, convulsive thresholds and dangers when mixed with alcohol!). This formulary is not exhaustive and may overlap with curriculum issues (*see* Chapter 7) and small group work (*see* Part 3).

Unfortunately the analogy with the formulary is inadequate in one essential respect. The drugs we use come prepared, packaged and guaranteed. Educational methods are not so conveniently prescribed. However, Figure 5.1 matches up educational aims with some of the methods described later in the chapter.

Educational aim	*Methods*
Exploration of attitudes	Problem case analysis, random case analysis, role-play, debate, Balint
Problem solving	Problem case analysis, brainstorming, buzz groups, critical incident, action learning
Communication skills	Micro-teaching using video material or role-play
Exploration of issues in depth	Debate, seminar, symposium, project, module
Methodology of learning (learning and study skills)	Action learning, teaching–learning group, project learning (library project or dissertation)
Presentation skills	Mini-lecture, micro-teaching, teaching–learning group
New factual learning	Lecture, symposium, seminar, project

Figure 5.1 Matching methods and aims.

The context of practical teaching

Group situations are most successful when:

- the group is working on problems and material which arise from the experience of its members – this ensures relevance and immediacy
- the group takes responsibility for its own learning needs – this ensures engagement and active learning
- the existing knowledge and experience of the learners are respected, explored and developed – this involves formative assessment (*see* Chapter 6) and not being afraid to search for gaps in knowledge
- participants are encouraged to explore techniques which allow them to get in touch with their own feelings (experiential learning)
- preparation and follow-up tasks supplement the teaching sessions to consolidate learning
- the group process is valued as well as the task with which it is engaged; how it works may be as vital as what it does (*see* Part 3)
- learning opportunities are recognized and exploited – this enhances the development of transferable skills and the generalization of learning from the particular to the principle (analysis and synthesis are complementary activities)
- a variety of teaching styles and modes of presentation are employed – this accommodates the variety of learning styles (*see* Chapter 4) which might be represented in the group
- a variety of assessment procedures is applied, again to motivate those with differing dominant learning styles
- there is an overall emphasis on what is done well.

The methods employed to put these principles into practice are listed below. A brief description of each is followed by a profile of its main educational qualities (positive and negative) and some guidelines for possible uses on the day-release course.

Menu of methods

Lecture

This continues to thrive despite criticism by educationalists. If the speaker is skilled, the subject matter appropriate and the audience committed, the lecture can still be the best way to convey specific information to a large group in a limited time.

PROFILE

Economical in terms of time, money and effort. It requires detailed preparation, good presentation skills and sensitivity to the needs of the audience, otherwise it can be boring and miss the mark. It is non-participatory, and learning tends to be passive.

USE

To present specific information about a topic in depth and to provide a synthesis or overview of a subject.

Symposium

This may refer to a conference or a publication. There is a demarcated subject and a number of appointed contributors deliver a variety of opinions on the subject, leading to a discussion. According to *The Shorter Oxford Dictionary* a symposium was originally a convivial meeting for drinking, conversation and intellectual entertainment.

PROFILE

Uses a variety of experts and complementary contributions. It can deal with a subject in depth, but is not very participatory and can be expensive, time consuming and complex.

USE

To give extensive coverage of a demarcated topic

Seminar

Originally this referred to a systematic study session under the direction of a teacher. More commonly it now refers to a group event based on discussion and resourced by someone with expertise in a given subject.

PROFILE

Participatory and flexible, and allows exploration of a subject in depth with one expert resource person.

USE

Allows input of information, an increase in the knowledge base and analysis and synthesis of a topic.

Debate

Derived from the Old French word for 'quarrel', it has come to mean a public discussion. As long as appropriate procedural rules are in place it provides an opportunity for teams of individuals to argue the merits of a proposition, without necessarily owning the opinions expressed. The outcome is frequently of subsidiary importance.

PROFILE

Deals with very specific issues of controversy. It is analytical and develops presentation skills, but can result in flippancy, point-scoring and competitiveness. The scope for participation is limited.

USE

To explore issues and attitudes, and develop presentation skills.

Buzz groups

Buzz groups are intended to combat inactivity in an audience by introducing some of the benefits of small group learning into audience-oriented teaching. At some stage in a presentation, those attending are invited to turn to a neighbour and share opinions and reactions for a short time. As an extension, the whole audience may be divided into small sub-groups for discussion. Feedback in the plenary setting is then usual. This provides stimulus for further input or clarification and may reduce the awkward silence which can be fatal to the question time.

PROFILE

Enhances engagement with a lecture and provokes ideas and questions: it is participatory but may be hard to manage.

Use

To break up a formal presentation and elicit audience response, and to ensure relevance in a presentation.

Mini-lecture

A short burst of input, fact or theory, in the course of a group activity aimed at stimulating discussion or linking up learning points. Participants may contribute their own ideas, thus increasing involvement with the material, introducing variety, distributing effort and responsibility, and developing presentation skills.

Profile

Diversifies proceedings and provides material which expands a group activity. Resource persons may operate in this way. It needs planning and preparation but is an economical way to use resources.

Use

Good for multiple skills training and group settings.

Specific task groups

These provide an efficient way of breaking down wide-ranging topics. Sub-groups are each allocated a topic to analyse and report back to plenary as a contribution towards a wider picture.

Profile

Self-resourced and economical, this method promotes active learning (i.e. members prepare topics themselves), peer learning (i.e. members learn from one another), and syndicate learning (i.e. division of labour and sharing of resources). It needs preparation and trainees often do not take each others' contributions seriously.

Use

To explore a broadly based topic, research the components and present them collaboratively. This method is good for multiple skills training and group settings.

EXAMPLE

Subject: health promotion and cancer. Introduction: theory, natural history of the diseases – screening. Specific tasks: 1 breast, 2 lung, 3 cervix, 4 large bowel.

Teaching–learning group

It is now fashionable to blur the distinction between teaching and learning, between expert and pupil. This technique is based on the observation that having to teach something to others is a very effective learning experience. One group designs a teaching programme to convey a given message to another group, and thus gain a full understanding of the content of the lesson. Roles are then reversed for a different topic. This helps establish teaching and learning as a transaction and develops presentation skills.

PROFILE

Active, syndicated, self-resourced and economical. Learning is reinforced by the teaching process.

USE

To explore demarcated topics, particularly for multiple skills training.

EXAMPLE: COMMISSIONING OF CARE

Group A: *'What is meant by fundholding?'* Group B: *'What is locality-based commissioning?'*

Brainstorming

This is a group technique which aims to generate a great variety and quantity of ideas in a short time. Given a problem, members are encouraged to suspend their critical faculty and produce any ideas and approaches to the question which occur to them. All are recorded unchallenged. The group then proceeds to elaborate, evaluate, discuss and resolve.

PROFILE

Participatory fun, encourages lateral thinking and contributes to group activity.

USE

To solve problems, make decisions and explore judgements or values.

EXAMPLE

John's practice is having problems starting a diabetic clinic. The main opponent seems to be the practice manager. Why? Think of as many reasons as you can, then recommend how he should proceed.

Action learning

This is based on the idea that the best way of learning is by doing, e.g. in the way that junior doctors learn minor surgery by 'watching one, doing one, teaching one'. Each member of a group can take on an identified problem or task, and report back regularly as he works through the issues towards solution or implementation. This is strongly advocated by Freire in his action/reflection cycle of learning.

PROFILE

It is active, with trainees engaging in a learning situation in real time, encountering and solving problems on the spot. It should be accompanied by reflection. It suits a variety of cognitive styles and requires preparation, supervision and time.

USE

To develop practical skills, e.g. clinical, communication and management skills, and to solve problems.

EXAMPLE

How do children cope with chronic illness? Next time you encounter a young person with diabetes/epilepsy/cerebral palsy/spina bifida explore with him or her its impact on everyday life.

Project-based learning

This is another learning-by-doing strategy. The trainees may choose the subject matter and direction, and are then required to produce a report on a topic or a plan which constitutes a solution to a problem. It has the advantages of stretching the trainee's abilities and encouraging the development of new skills. It demands initiative, creativity and organizational abilities. Learning is active. It may resemble the specific task group if projects are based on a common theme. Sharing of project outcomes, with commentary by an expert on that area, can be a useful way of teaching the essentials of broadly based subjects like health education or management.

PROFILE

Suitable for a variety of learning styles, the learner works at his own pace and in his own way, accumulating, analysing and presenting his own data. Presentation is oral or in writing. It needs supervision, assessment and time.

USE

For multiple (transferable) skills development, syndicating and the methodology of learning.

EXAMPLE

Think of a practical change in the procedures of your practice you would like to introduce. Draw up a plan for implementing it.

Modular learning

Modules are units of education and have been called 'quantities of learning to be achieved' (RCGP, 1990).

Many themes seem too wide for adequate treatment in a day-release course. Such themes can be reduced to component parts which are then presented separately over a period of time to build a composite picture. This is fashionable in distance learning in continuing medical education, and where participants can only come together periodically. Some Scottish schemes employ this technique widely. A variation is to approach the theme using a variety of opportunities and settings, leading to a plenary session for further input and task setting, with later reinforcement and follow-up. Many schemes have set-piece modules on central themes in which a lot of resources are invested, a variety of learning/teaching opportunities and techniques are employed, and a range of educational aims are realized and evaluated.

PROFILE

The timespan fosters involvement and progressive learning. The variety of approaches accommodates different learning styles, and allows generalization and reinforcement of learning. It is time and resource intensive and needs careful planning.

USE

For dealing with extensive topics or linked themes, in a block of time or over a series of sessions. Good for multiple skills learning.

EXAMPLE

Module on substance abuse. *Aims:* to explore current theories of addiction; the effects of substance abuse on the patient, the family and society; the GP response; managing acute toxicity; prevention; to create a practice protocol involving community resources. *Methods:* reading list; practice audit; tutorial with trainer; symposium; group work; follow-up assessment.

Case discussion

As a formal or informal educational method, this is indispensable. Rooted in real life and in the personal experience of the learners involved, posing real questions for practical solutions yet flexible enough to range beyond the immediate, it has many characteristics of an ideal problem-based learning tool. It can employ features of role-play, micro-teaching, group work and critical incident. It may focus on issues of clinical content, process, communication, decision making and consultation technique, especially when based on a video-recording of a real or simulated case. The principal difficulties include lack of focus, ineffective use of time and avoidance of confrontation. Two important variants are stalwarts of day-release courses.

In *random case analysis* the records of a sequence of cases from a surgery are produced without selection and presented for a review of aspects of management. This can reveal gaps in the trainee's learning and bring up issues which might never have been identified by examining selected cases. It resembles the simulated surgery.

Problem case analysis brings the varied perspectives and expertise of the group to bear on problems which the trainee has encountered. Such an exercise should be planned well in advance. When used in conjunction with follow-up discussion, there are features of action learning or Balint-type activity in which support, reflection and problem solving are valuable components.

PROFILE

Reality based, versatile, relevant and economical.

USE

To explore attitudes, decision making, problem solving and clinical skills – spontaneously or after planning – and to feed group work.

The Balint group

A familiar activity in continuing education, the Balint group can contribute greatly to the day-release course. It shares features with problem case analysis. The focus of the Balint method is firmly on the doctor and his awareness of his own feelings about an unfolding case that is presenting challenges, rather than on the clinical content of the case. It is a useful way of helping trainees who may be sceptical about process group work (and sensitivity training, *see* Chapter 1) to focus on their own feelings and attitudes, identify the feelings of others and be aware of a symbolic level to the consultation.

PROFILE

Reality based, versatile, relevant and economical. It requires a lot of time to explore properly the benefits of serial discussion of cases which are evolving over a period of time.

USE

To explore attitudes, feelings, empathy and problem solving. Peer learning and group work provide support with difficult situations.

Critical incident

This refers to the discussion and analysis of a particular event, based on real life: a dilemma, problem or crisis described by one participant. The event should be typical rather than extraordinary as what appears to be mundane is rendered critical through analysis (Tripps, 1993). The RCGP report on critical incident refers to it as significant event audit (RCGP, 1996). The group's task is to examine or speculate about the possible background to the incident, the feelings and thoughts which might be experienced by the various parties involved, and the kind of dialogue which might ensue. They then suggest a variety of possible outcomes and reflect on what has been learnt. This gives participants a safe method of exploring new ways of thinking and feeling, which may lead easily to role-play.

PROFILE

Reality based, relevant, analytical, experiential and allows skill development in a secure setting. It requires little preparation.

USE

For experiential or affective learning, and to develop empathy, insight, analytical and problem-solving skills. It is a useful way of learning how to respond to threatening situations.

EXAMPLE

Your receptionist phones during surgery to tell you that the next patient on your list was very abusive to her on arrival. How do you respond to this situation? Discuss in small groups and prepare a role-play. Create guidelines for reception staff on how to respond to difficult patients.

Role-play

There is a consensus among educationalists that this is a very valuable technique for teaching interpersonal skills and exploring attitudes to situations. These are difficult to approach with less experientially based methods. Role-play works best when it arises naturally in the process of one-to-one teaching or group work. Characters are allocated and given an outline of the situation so that a scenario can be enacted. As confidence in role-play grows, its potential as a learning tool expands. The participants can put themselves in the shoes of a patient (or other character) and thereby gain insight into how he or she might feel or act. Role reversal is a useful extension. Those playing the doctor and patient change places and rerun the scenario, thereby providing opportunities for the participants to change their perceptions and develop empathy. A further refinement is the use of *simulated patients:* actors (or people capable of acting) who have a relatively full script of a patient's problem. This can be rerun with different trainees adopting the role of the doctor. Experienced actors are good at giving feedback about what the transaction felt like from the patient's perspective. In the group situation it is important for onlookers to be sensitive to the process. Unexpected levels of feeling may be generated in the participants. It is essential that there is *'de-roling'* at the end of the exercise, with feedback or some symbolic action whereby each player is permitted consciously to relinquish the adopted roles and resume their normal personas. Interdisciplinary learning may also be approached in this way, with role-playing, team meetings or case conferences.

PROFILE

Experiential, participatory, flexible and analytical. Replay, role reversal and feedback allow exploration of alternative processes or outcomes. It can appear threatening, at first, and is often regarded as contrived. It may need preparation but it can also be spontaneous.

USE

To develop communication skills, empathy, insight and problem solving; to explore attitudes.

EXAMPLE

Scenario for role-play: a case conference on child abuse (details supplied). What are the issues for each person round the table? What feelings might this situation arouse in each? What about the child and the family?

Triadic teaching

A relatively new word for the collection, but a technique of long standing in vocational training. The triad refers to the three key participants but, curiously, there is often a fourth party (the facilitator whose job is to identify learning opportunities). The three players are the Subject, presenting a real, unresolved problem; the Listener, who reflects the content and feelings of the subject; and the Observer who, through active listening, observes the transaction.

PROFILE

As for critical incident.

USE

To develop active listening skills and sensitivity to the affective content of a transaction.

Problem-based learning

This is more an educational philosophy than an educational tool. It is an approach to curriculum planning and execution which employs group methods to explore and research the ramifications of a practical problem statement, and reflect on what is learnt in the process. It is treated in greater depth in Chapter 8.

Portfolio-based learning

A method of organizing learning, like an educational CV, rather than a teaching tool. The portfolio contains accounts of learning exercises undertaken, projects or modules completed, evidence of educational attainment and anything that contributes towards the learner's personal professional development. It is increasingly used in continuing education because of its longitudinal quality. With the prospect of extended vocational training, educative experience in multiple situations and modular examinations it will have an increasing place in vocational training. It is the subject of a major College report (RCGP, 1994).

Evidence-based learning

Another 'new wine in old wineskins' topic and more fully discussed in Chapter 14. Our medical culture has always sought to be evidence based. The work of Archie Cochrane and David Sackett has given impetus to the need to take account of empirical evidence in the development of thinking on any given topic. The avalanche of medical publications has been recognized as a major learning problem. This can only be addressed through an analytical approach to the quality and source of information with special emphasis on the outcomes of controlled trials and the development of meta-analysis technique. This has given rise to the Cochrane Collaboration, various databases derived from syndicated study of the international medical literature and publication of these in ways which are authoritative, updated and accessible. This evidence-based culture is permeating all professional training. It is embodied in the critical reading components of the MRCGP examination and is an essential feature of exam preparation.

Micro-teaching

This is a way of analysing complex behaviour like communication and consultation. It typically employs the video-recording of a learning exercise, which is then viewed in a tutorial or group setting with safeguards relating to confidentiality and 'Pendleton's Rules'. The behaviour is broken down into component parts and discussed, teaching points are identified and feedback is given. This is time consuming but leads to greater understanding.

PROFILE

Personalized, analytical and experiential. It needs preparation and safeguards. It is time consuming and can feel threatening.

USE

For skills training.

Video-teaching

The camcorder is now standard teaching equipment. Trainers are required actively to use VCRs with their trainee. In addition to examination requirements its main applications are for recording cases for subsequent discussion, micro-teaching and distance learning. In the day-release course, there are the added dynamic factors of group activity, the facility to observe and analyse group process issues, and to engage in role-play. Such equipment should be available at the day-release course venue. Consent and confidentiality are important. The technicalities of using the camera are best learnt from a competent audio-visual technician and by gaining experience with a particular model. Badly made videos are distracting.

The use of pre-recorded material is an important teaching resource. Much high-quality material is available through pharmaceutical companies, charities, national

TV networks, various distance learning programmes and local medical libraries. The videocassette now constitutes an extension to medical literature and may be used like any other library material.

PROFILE

It is flexible but requires safeguards in preparation and use, and some find it threatening. Confidentiality is important. Playback at an individual's or group's own pace can make it time consuming. The initial capital outlay is significant.

USE

To encourage group discussion, to record and analyse group work, and for skills training. It is also required for the summative assessments.

Exercise 11

How many of the above educational techniques did you use in the past term?

How might you diversify this?

Scenario: What's going on?

(A further discussion between Meeke and Best)

Best: *Well, you're through your first term. How is it so far?*

Meeke: *It's gone very smoothly. The trainees are a good bunch. They're beginning to read, they say they look forward to Thursday afternoons, all the speakers turned up at the right times and the term flew by at an incredible rate. The trainers' workshops are producing an assessment package. After all I have heard about how time consuming and difficult course organizing is, I'm wondering where I'm going wrong. I'm not supposed to enjoy it, am I?*

Best: *Of course you are! Don't look for trouble. What do you think has made it good so far?*

Meeke: *I think I'm learning a lot. The trainees are very knowledgeable – they know more than I do about clinical medicine, but they often can't see the wood for the trees and I'm enjoying the discovery that I have a clearer overview of things than they have. I can feel my confidence growing. I'm even beginning to enjoy my general practice* work more because I'm looking at it differently. Problem situations have become things to discuss with the trainees. I often think I'm learning more than the trainees are! And when I find an area which I'm weak on, I can arrange a session, get a speaker and fill in my own gaps.

Best: *That's good, as long as you remember that the day-release is not entirely for your benefit! But an interested teacher who is himself growing is likely to have better results. Also, a teacher who knows what he doesn't know is less likely to fall into the trap of being dogmatic and relying on didactic methods. He's more likely to involve the students in the learning process and employ a diversity of teaching and learning styles. A friend of mine says that to be a good teacher you don't have to know very much yourself – you only have to know how to ask questions and where to go to discover the answers. I believe Socrates didn't teach much, he used provocative questions and let the pupils teach each other by discussion and discovery.*

Meeke: *Didn't he end up getting bumped off for corrupting the minds of the youth?*

Best: *Touché! Merely a sign of his effectiveness, and I've yet to hear of a martyred course organizer. Let's move on to the rocky bits. You had a few early on and I'm sure it's not all plain sailing. You're uneasy about something.*

Meeke: *Yes. The other day the secretary asked if I had next term's programme ready yet. I suddenly realized that I was coasting towards the end of term on the strength of what had been arranged, and I hadn't looked beyond Christmas. Now I have the prospect of spending the festive season sorting things out for January, February and March at a time when nobody's at work, and if I can get them on the phone they're in no mood for discussing a plan for some February afternoon.*

Best: *That's the down side of organizing. You're liable to find that it intrudes on your own time – evenings, weekends and holidays. It's hard to find any time during the ordinary working day to plan and make arrangements. You have to live in the future all the time, keeping an eye on the months ahead. You'll find that life speeds up and terms flash by because you're always meeting deadlines. So, what've you done?*

Meeke: *I had another panic attack! I decided to start on next term's programme that same evening. It was the most dismal experience yet. I didn't even know how long the term was supposed to be because I couldn't find out when Easter comes. In the end I looked up last year's programme, decided on a few topics, and thought of some suitable speakers for them – but almost everyone I phoned was out. I filled one slot and decided to call it a night.*

Best: *Don't worry. It's a mistake to get too focused on the programme as an end in itself – it's not the measure of your success. It's purely a vehicle for your ideas. Of course there are things which have to be written down as fixed points in the term. To some extent the programme writes itself – starting and finishing dates, meetings for the whole scheme, that sort of thing. You could have a perfectly valid educational package based on an otherwise blank programme. An equally valid one might look like a secondary school timetable. What counts is the values, themes, quality of resource people and how much the trainees get involved in the process of learning. A month or a term programme is meaningless unless seen in the context of the overall training process. Now, I suggest you forget about your programme for the time being and spend a while writing down your statements of principles, like an election manifesto – your hopes, plans, ideas and intentions. Look at your own and past programmes critically and list their strengths and weaknesses. For example, looking through your programme I see you have relied heavily on clinical talks by hospital consultants. To what extent were the trainees involved in selecting, participating and assessing? What variety of educational methods did you deploy during the term? Could you have drawn on a wider variety of resource persons? In other words, what would you like your trainees to learn, how and from whom? If you make out lists along these lines, your programme will emerge more easily, not just this time but every time.*

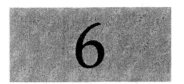

Assessment in vocational training

Introduction

'Most teachers are attracted into education not because they fantasized in childhood about assessing educational outcomes and processes, but because they want to teach. Assessment tends to be accepted as a necessary part of the educational package.' (Anonymous course organizer)

It could be said that assessment is to education as management is to clinical practice. Why do we not remember Dr Finlay doing any practice administration, or Miss Jean Brodie doing any assessments? The simple answer is that they are fictional (not that they are both Scots!). Assessment is high on the agenda of vocational training for a variety of reasons, some of them educational:

- educators wish to refine their educational activities
- learners wish to be validated at the end of the educational process
- society demands an assurance of competence as a product of professional training
- politicians and administrators demand evidence of value for money in a shrinking economy
- the fashion has shifted to focus on assessment as the key to movement in the educational triangle so that it becomes an educational cycle that actually revolves.

These differing concerns would be relatively easy to reconcile if there were a clear consensus on the aims and content of training. Unfortunately, the nature of general practice makes it difficult to achieve such a consensus.

Assessment is therefore a challenging concept. As the educational overseer of vocational training you have an essential role in co-ordinating and advising on educational assessment. You should be familiar with the methods used in the training practice and hospital posts, in addition to those appropriate to the day-release course setting. All of these have much in common.

Like many aspects of professional practice, assessment will not flourish if it is approached reluctantly or with resentment. Actively managed, it can motivate learners and aid learning. '*The assessment system is the most potent factor influencing student learning behaviour*' (Newble and Entwhistle, 1986).

Assessment of competence

'*Assessment is an integral part of the educational process*' (Merrison, 1975)

Professional competence implies more than a body of knowledge and skills. There is a poor correlation between what people know and what they do. There is an inverse relationship between the things we most value in professional practice and the ease of measuring them, as illustrated by Einstein's statement: '*Not everything that counts can be counted and not everything that can be counted counts.*' This might be described as the 'inverse core law' – matters central to our discipline are less accessible and less easily assessed than those which are peripheral.

In assessing professional practice, therefore, we encounter a conflict between relevance and rigour, as enshrined in the concepts of validity and reliability. Validity is the extent to which the method of assessment really tests what it is designed to test (JCPTGP, 1995). Reliability is the consistency with which it does so. For example, examinations are reliable but are not a very valid way to test the attainment of aims such as competence. Observation, on the other hand, is a most valid way of assessing competence, but there are technical difficulties in doing this comprehensively and objectively enough to be reliable (RCGP, 1988).

Much education has what sociologists call 'face validity': it is deemed to be so obviously right that there is no need to think about it any more (Tait, 1987). This is the basis of the apprenticeship style of training – the candidate serves his time and is accredited accordingly. General practice vocational training was established in this mould as an extension of the idea of the pre-registration year.

Until recently the Joint Committee on Postgraduate Training for General Practice (JCPTGP) issued a certificate of completion of vocational training to any candidate who submitted evidence of satisfactory completion of each of the stages of training (forms VTR1 by the practice trainer and VTR2 for each hospital post). The criteria of satisfaction constituted a problem of legal definition. This gave rise to the need for a standardized national framework for assessing trainees in the UK, in line with EU directives.

There appear to be three main issues:

1 educational values demand that an educational process has some worth or validity. In the absence of criteria, what does validity mean?

2 the place of examinations in professional training is controversial. Effective assessment systems imply a failure rate

3 pressure is mounting to ensure that certification refers to ensuring competence rather than completion.

Assessment, therefore, is about identifying, defining and measuring criteria related to process and outcome.

There is a resemblance here to the audit cycle. However, there are two concepts that need to be distinguished: *summative assessment* which relates to outcome and *formative assessment* which relates to the processes (a form of educational audit). They have complementary functions. When formative assessment takes on summative features the result is continuous assessment.

Summative assessment

The time-honoured educational system erected 'gates' at crucial stages of the process, each constituting some kind of endpoint. Those who got through were successes, those who did not were failures and had to seek some other path or drop out. Summative assessment is controversial at all educational levels. It tends to emphasize rigour at the expense of relevance, the validity *v* reliability question. The concept of endpoint assessment does not contribute essentially to the professional growth of the individual. Summative assessment is further considered in Chapter 7.

'The purpose of summative assessment is protection of patients and the regulation of the profession.' (JCPTGP, 1995)

Formative assessment

'The purpose of formative assessment is education.' (JCPTGP, 1992)

Formative assessment is a more or less continuous process whereby teacher and learner interact to identify and explore learning needs and develop strategies for fulfilling them. There is an increasing awareness that trainees in general practice are adult learners rather than advanced students. Accordingly there is an emphasis on autonomous and continuing learning. Trainees are encouraged to become involved in the assessment of their own progress in conjunction with their trainer and hospital consultants. There is also an increase in the use of strategies to enable trainees to identify their own learning needs. The purpose of formative assessment is to identify areas of weakness which require special attention. Formative assessment is designed for relevance, perhaps at the expense of rigour. Its focus on the process of learning is clearly related to the quality of outcome.

A survey of UK regional assessment activities carried out by the Vocational Training Working Group of the RCGP (Gambril et al., 1991) showed that:

- all regions were actively involved in stimulating and encouraging systematic assessment during the final trainee (registrar) year
- formative assessment during the hospital period of training was much less well developed, although widespread local initiatives were proceeding
- there was a lack of regional and national criteria for evaluation of the reliability of the various assessments applied.

Such lack of uniformity in assessment reflects the state of vocational training in most dimensions. Paradoxically, one of the historical strengths of vocational training for general practice in Great Britain and Ireland is the autonomy of regions and local schemes, promoting diversity and new ideas. This has resulted in the development of an increasing range of assessment methods. In 1993, the JCPTGP included format-ive assessment among the minimum criteria to be met by training practice and hos-pital posts.

The ACO working party report on assessment (Sackin et al., 1988) is essential reading for all involved in trainee assessment. Of particular value is its section on the principles of assessment.

Principles of assessment

Professionalism

Much professional assessment goes on informally in the course of vocational train-ing. It is based on a mixture of gut feelings and observation of an individual's reason-ing, presentation skills and interaction with peers. These observations are useful only if they are recorded, fed back to the trainee and used as a basis for structuring change. The fact that they defy rigorous measurement should not diminish their validity. In the words of Gronlund (1988): 'Observational data play an important role in evaluating performance skills and in evaluating those affective outcomes that are reflected in the individual's typical behaviour.'

Trainee-centredness

Trainees should be involved in assessing their own progress. If both trainee and course organizer share responsibility for achieving the aims of the course, the need for conflict is minimized.

Content of assessment

This should cover the whole range of needs for becoming a principal in general practice: knowledge, skills and attitudes. Various instruments (checklists, computer software etc) are available to ensure that the necessary areas are covered. (A further dimension is to ensure that they have actually been learned.)

Use of different assessment methods

Learning behaviour is complex and is profoundly influenced by the assessment methods employed (Newble and Entwhistle, 1986) (*see* the discussion of learning styles in Chapter 5). To foster balanced learning it is advisable to use the widest variety of assessment methods and to collate assessment from as many sources as possible, including consultants and trainers. The question of who should be responsible for collating such data is open to debate, but the course organizer is probably best placed to do so (Hayden, 1996).

Good communication

Effective assessment – integrating hospital, practice and day-release components – requires clear lines of communication. Confidentiality can be a problem. The trainers' workshop is a useful forum for discussing problems which arise in relation to trainees. However, a trainee should not be identified or discussed in the presence of people who are not personally responsible for his current progress without his consent or involvement. The trainee should own his progress record and be involved in its evolution.

Methods of assessment

The following methods are more fully described in the ACO report and in many articles in the *Journal of the Association of Course Organizers*, especially Volume 2, No 1

(1986) and Volume 4, No 1(1988), and its offspring journal, *Education for General Practice.*

The multiple choice question paper (MCQ)

PROFILE

Has high reliability but is very limited for assessing general practice competence. Sampling of knowledge is random. Although difficult to set, it is simple to mark.

USE

Because it focuses on overall scores rather than problem areas, it has limited use in formative assessment. It is most useful at the start of each course to screen for gross defects in clinical knowledge which may then be rectified. It is also useful in preparing for the examinations.

The modified essay question paper (MEQ)

PROFILE

Reliable and valid, it can reproducibly test knowledge and attitudinal areas, and some skills. Unfortunately it is difficult to set and mark.

USE

Used as a baseline and recurrently to cover a wide range of situations; as a basis for group discussion; and for MRCGP exam preparation.

The objective structured clinical examination (OSCE)

PROFILE

Measures components of clinical competence in a way that is more valid and reliable than traditional clinical exams. The skills and competences to be tested are identified, and clinical 'stations' are devised to demonstrate them in action in the presence of an observer who has a preset marking schedule. Other stations may be information based, e.g. a photograph or a report of an investigation. Routinely used in many regions.

ADVANTAGES

Versatility, validity for general practice assessment, immediacy of feedback on performance through active participation by resource persons, and fairly high degree of reliability.

DISADVANTAGES

Logistics (and expense) and difficulty of devising tests which explore certain areas such as beliefs and values. It is incorporated into the membership examination of the Irish College, where the main problem is that it is not a highly discriminating test. Since the MICGP is the Irish national certification exam, this lack of sensitivity may actually be an advantage.

USE

For formative assessment and on-the-spot feedback. Its complexity means that it can only be used about once a year. It is very educative for all involved, not just the candidates.

Simulated surgery

PROFILE

This resembles a role-played MEQ, using experienced actors to simulate the kind of problem sequences that might present during a surgery. It has the advantage of detailed feedback from the 'patient' perspective, but requires a lot of preparation of 'stations' and detailed briefing of actors.

USE

Dependent on local availability of experienced role-players. Actors de-role at the end, giving feedback to candidates, providing an excellent opportunity for learning insight. Useful for formative assessment of clinical and interpersonal skills. It has now found a limited place in the MRCGP exam as an alternative to the video component.

Continuous trainee-centred assessment (CTCA)

PROFILE

The day-to-day observations of trainer and trainee are recorded so that both can identify needs, set goals and assess progress. It can be modified for use on the day-release course. Learning needs for the group are identified and recorded, priorities are agreed between the group and the course organizer. The group takes responsibility for ensuring that these learning needs are met. It is well described in the ACO report.

USE

Regularly, especially in the training practice, to provide a cumulative record of goals (set and met) and to assess the course.

Project work

PROFILE

Much course work in vocational training is based on action learning through audit-related activities and minor projects. Many schemes entail a major project assessed by the trainee group itself or by invited resource persons. These are valuable educational exercises which say much about those undertaking them. May need to provide advice and direction. A method of evaluating projects is shown in Chapter 14. It is now an essential feature of the summative assessment examination, where it takes the form of an audit.

USE

To develop skills in information gathering, library work, problem solving and presentation. All project work should be assessed and recorded.

Random case analysis (RCA)

PROFILE

This is an example of how a routine teaching method functions equally as an assessment tool. Trainees are asked to bring all the case notes from their last surgery for discussion of randomly selected cases along group work lines.

USE

To explore gaps in perception and for decision making; it is a much-used day-release course activity. The ACO report recommends the following list of options:

- concentrate on the overt problems
- tackle undeclared problems
- relate previously identified learning needs to the case under discussion
- test the trainees' knowledge, skills and attitudes against previously identified needs
- identify problems as they arise, and perhaps discuss them at a later session.

Problem case analysis (PCA)

This may be used in much the same way, and can sometimes explore issues in greater depth.

The use of video for assessment

Originally used universally as a tool of formative assessment, it has been incorporated into both major examinations (*see* Chapter 7). Proper equipment is essential for training practices. Its use by course organizers is mainly in the analysis of recorded consultations. The purpose is to evaluate the ability of members of the group to appreciate what is going on in a consultation and how their analytic skills are developing. Much useful information, including the General Medical Council (GMC) guidelines on confidentiality and consent, is given in Field (1995).

Assessment packs

These are produced in many regions. Good examples are available from Yorkshire and Leicester Regions. They are mostly concerned with the training practice situation and the assessment of competences by the trainers. They include the use of joint consultation, analysis of video-recorded consultations and audit of aspects of the trainee's work.

Mock MRCGP Exam

PROFILE

A full-scale replica of the membership examination, it is a feature of the Northern Ireland scheme where there is widespread acceptance of the MRCGP as a rite of passage at the end of training. It is demanding and expensive to mount, but involvement of the trainer workshops in setting and marking the papers and oral examining are considered valuable by all concerned.

USE

As a one-off trial run for registrars, some months before the membership exam; to prepare for summative assessment (although it also has some formative features).

Psychometric tests

PROFILE

These are questionnaires which explore personality traits or cognitive style, based on psychological testing methods. They are validated statistically on standard populations, including medical students and doctors. They are usually easily administered, and marking is automated or by template. It may be expensive where testing materials are copyrighted and restricted to authorized users. They do not seem to be widely used in vocational training in the UK.

Examples include:

- FIRO-B; 16PF personality test; used in Exeter VTS to promote individual awareness and as a basis for group work
- Learning style questionnaire, a tool which indicates areas of cognitive strength or weakness (Honey and Mumford, 1992)
- Myers-Briggs Type Indicator; used in Northern Ireland VTS. May help with insight into cognitive style, areas of special ability or vulnerability and career guidance
- S-SDLRS, a questionnaire which explores self-directed learning (Bligh, 1993)
- Various attitudinal questionnaires as used in Sheffield VTS.

USE

Usually as a one-off, not strictly speaking for assessment, although profiling may have formative value in highlighting learning difficulties. It can give learners insight into their areas of difficulty and provide the impetus to practise compensatory mechanisms.

The structure of trainee assessment

The assessment of the trainee group is a continuous process. The concept of three terms or two semesters in the year provides a framework of assessment points, e.g. start of year, end of terms and end of year, with mid-term options if necessary. No timetable has yet been adopted nationally, although it is much debated.

The initial assessment is useful for stocktaking, setting goals and planning the curriculum, and may be done in conjunction with the trainer; the use of multiple methods can identify major learning needs.

The end of term assessment should consist of an interview with appraisal and a review of all written assessment records. It may be worth employing a third party to take part in assessing the whole process, including evaluation of the course.

The end of year assessment is useful for those who are going to return the following year, and for the course organizer who is reviewing his year's work.

It is more difficult to carry out structured assessment of trainees in SHO posts since many are not formally linked to the VTS from the start. Hospitals are required to have a policy of regular appraisal of SHOs (RCP, 1997) (*see* Part 4).

Keeping assessment records

Both the RCGP and ACO reports on assessment recommend that recording should be:

- regular (continuing)
- systematic (structured in some way)
- open (shared and owned by trainee and assessor)
- written in some sort of proforma or log-book.

Maintaining such records ensures that learning opportunities are not overlooked and constitutes evidence of work done. This can be important in those cases where certification is in doubt or has to be withheld. Unfortunately there is a strong tendency for paper to accumulate, and this can quench enthusiasm.

The confidentiality and ownership of the material by the trainee, in the form of a log-book, are important features of recording. A portfolio of assessments, projects, audits and other specific exercises may accumulate through the hospital and trainee years and contribute to assessment. Portfolio learning, as it is called, is a developing area of professional practice. On the wider educational scene it forms the basis of the credit accumulation transfer system (CATS).

Assessing the course

It is perhaps a false dichotomy to distinguish between the assessment of trainees and the assessment of the course. According to Brooks (1986): *'Although the distinction can be helpful in practice, the two are inextricably combined. The trainee's feelings about the course tell the course organizer a great deal about the trainee.'*

What the trainees think of us and our courses may need a good deal of interpretation. However, as Bahrami (1989) pointed out, the course organizer is much less subject to assessment than the trainee or trainer. We therefore have a professional responsibility to assess our own efforts (Ball and Siegel, 1995). Our complex job description suggests that many areas might be subjected to quality control. Since the day-release course is at the core of our concern, this must be the first area of evaluation and there are a number of possible ways.

Continuing evaluation

A short questionnaire is completed by the trainees at the end of the day-release course session. Information is sought about their perception of the content, presentation and relevance, and new learning outcomes are identified. This implies that the trainees have some idea of the educational aims; if you do not have any stated aims it is difficult to assess the quality of your efforts. If the invited speaker's contribution is apparently pointless, this may be because he or she was not properly briefed by the course organizer, which is a reflection on them both. Of course the written comments can also help assess the trainee's performance as a learner during the session. It takes time at the end of the session for the course organizer to examine, collate, interpret and learn from the report sheets. This process can make a valuable contribution to curriculum development as new input, approaches and resource persons are tried, tested and changed.

Many types of report form are in common use or can be devised (Gibbs *et al.*, 1988). Typical examples are reproduced in Figures 6.1 and 6.2. Different types of learning exercise require different proformas for evaluation.

Date	Subject 1	Subject 2	Subject 3
Title/speaker Relevance to my needs (score 1–5)			
Quality of content (score 1–5)			
Quality of presentation (score 1–5)			
What I liked about the session			
Suggest change (specify)			
Open comments/suggestions			
Give score 1–5 plus analytical comment and return to course organizer/secretary			

Figure 6.1 Evaluation form, Northern Ireland.

Interviews with trainees

It is customary in many schemes for the course organizer to conduct individual interviews with the trainees periodically, to set goals and give assessment, guidance ('pastoral' and otherwise) and feedback (*see* Chapter 13). It also gives the trainees a chance to make suggestions and comments about the course.

There can be problems arising from a 'collusion of cosiness', a tacit mutual agreement not to rock the boat. Trainees are likely to feel too inhibited to give much criticism of the course when they are face-to-face with their course organizer. Evaluation carried out at a year-end interview can suffer from the drawbacks of summative assessment, without the safeguards. There is little point in eliciting uninhibited feedback from individuals who have no further investment in the process and when it is too late to take corrective action. This problem is avoided where assessment is carried out by a trained and supportive third party, as described below.

Please circle 0–3 closest to your opinion

Subject _____ Date _____

Facilitator _____

3	Strongly agree/Disagree
2	Agree/Disagree
1	Partially agree/Disagree
0	Don't know/Not applicable

Please feel free to write your reasons on the sheet

	Agree				Disagree		
The suggested preparation was appropriate	3	2	1	0	1	2	3
There was useful discussion	3	2	1	0	1	2	3
Meeting relevant to general practice	3	2	1	0	1	2	3
I have been stimulated to think again about this topic	3	2	1	0	1	2	3
Facilitator was well prepared	3	2	1	0	1	2	3
This meeting is worth repeating	3	2	1	0	1	2	3

Suggestions for improvement:

Other subjects which should be in the programme:

General comments

Figure 6.2 Evaluation form, South-West Scotland.

Peer visiting

Styles (1986) suggested that day-release course sessions should be observed periodically by two peers of the course organizer from another region. Views would also be sought from the trainee group. This would be supplemented by a pre-visit questionnaire and a constructive follow-up report. Styles also listed quality criteria for a course organizer – an important pre-requisite where the subject of assessment is not so much the course as the course organizer (*see* Chapter 3).

Trainer assessment of the course

Brooks (1986) described a method of managing the end-of-term evaluation. A representative of the trainer's workshop carries out a similar role to that of the visiting course organizer as described above, and discusses his observations with the course organizer who is being assessed.

Annual report

The production of an annual report by each course organizer in a scheme is a well-established activity for self-assessment and peer learning. It helps brief the regional director about the educational activities of the day-release course, and perhaps wider issues as well. Crabbe (1986) discussed the possibility of regional, and even national, standardization. In its simplest form the report might list and describe the educational activities of the year, with a statement of aims and a discussion of problems, innovations and plans for future development. This provides a useful basis for group discussion at regional course organizer meetings.

Postscript

The proper use of all formative assessment methods should be based on an educational understanding which safeguards the dignity and autonomy of the learner, promotes openness and reciprocity, encourages continued learning, recognizes the limitations of the underlying assumptions, and takes account of the resource and administrative implications.

Any programme of assessment must allow for the organic unity of the educational triangle (*see* Figure 6.3).

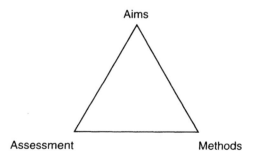

Figure 6.3 The educational triangle.

You cannot just break off the 'Assessment' corner and deal with it in isolation. Assessment – of the trainee and the course – may be seen as one of the common threads linking education, group work and management, the course organizer's three main disciplines.

Assessment acronyms and abbreviations

The growth of local initiatives which receive wider attention has given rise to a stamp-collector's problem: identification of acronyms and abbreviations. A short identification chart has become necessary.

ACCESS	Assessment of Clinical Competence European Study Syndicate (a consultation assessment programme developed jointly by Leicester and Amsterdam)
CATS	Credit accumulation transfer system
CRQ	Critical reading question paper
CTCA	Continuous trainee-centred assessment
CV	Curriculum vitae
EMQ	Extended matching questions (a variation on the MCQ form)
MRCGP	Membership examination of the Royal College of General Practitioners
MARS	Mutually agreed reporting system
MCQ	Multiple choice question paper
MEQ	Modified essay question paper
MRS	Manchester Rating Scale
OSCE	Objective structured clinical examination
PCA	Problem case analysis
PEP	Phased evaluation programme
PROP	Progress recording, observation, planning
PMP	Patient management problem
RCA	Random case analysis
SAQ	Short answer questionnaire
TRAD	Trainee rolling assessment diary
UKRA	United Kingdom Regional Advisers' Assessment examination (the summative assessment)

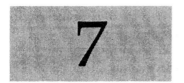

7

Summative assessment

'Assessment of VT is a subject that engenders strong feelings amongst educationalists, those being educated and representatives of the service element of the discipline.' (JCPTGP, 1993)

Introduction

The examination system entered a transitional phase in 1996 with the introduction of extensive changes to the MRCGP exam and the implementation of a new, nationwide test of minimum competence – the Summative Assessment or UK Regional Advisers' Assessment.

The early experience of this transition has, for many, confirmed a sense of foreboding. Years of work by the ACO had succeeded in establishing formative assessment as the preferred educational approach to the point where, in 1993, it became a minimum educational criterion for all training posts. Formative assessment was compatible with the routine tasks and rhythm of the practice training year. Although time and labour intensive, it held the promise of raising standards across the whole spectrum of training posts, trainers and training practices (and COs).

At a time when resources were under considerable pressure it was realized that, inevitably, the burden of administering the additional exam system would fall to the minority of GPs who had educational credentials. This coincided with an era of unprecedented change in the delivery of general practice services and the triple role of clinical practice, teaching and examining was daunting. At the same time there emerged what came to be known as the recruitment crisis in general practice. There was a quantitative (and possibly qualitative) decline in applicants for schemes, combined with a reduction in the number of those proceeding to take up definitive posts in general practice. Not surprisingly, this complex of issues became confused in people's perceptions, resulting in hostility towards any change.

Course organizers were aware of the 'strong feelings' acknowledged by the Joint Committee in 1993. These found a focus in the new summative assessment exam. Its opponents could claim that there are two competing approaches – the formative one, based on educational principle and the optimal use of existing resources, and the summative one based on an administrative, consumerist and political analysis. In this they reflected the feelings of trainees (especially registrars) concerning a double hurdle to be faced and the possibility that failure could constitute an absolute bar to entry to general practice. It also represented the feelings of the trainers and course organizers about a process which entailed a lot of extra effort, much of it considered tedious, which would dominate the other educational objectives in the busy schedule of practice-based training.

Alternative introduction

Since the RCGP Quality Initiative (RCGP, 1985) there has been a growing debate about the value of the Joint Committee's Certificate of Satisfactory Completion of Vocational Training as the definitive ticket for entry into general practice. Concerns were raised by college examiners that even though not all trainees undertook the membership exam a substantial proportion of those elected to do so were failing, some by a wide margin. The JCPTGP, therefore, appointed a working party to 'consider methods of ensuring a doctor's competence to become a principal in the NHS and to make recommendations' (JCPTGP, 1987).

A number of issues needed to be addressed:

1 What are the desirable attributes of a doctor entering general practice other than endurance through a tough three-year programme?
2 Can the VTR1 and VTR2 certificates (issued by practice- and hospital-based trainers respectively, on satisfactory *completion* of each post) be relied upon to ensure the attainment of a satisfactory level of *competence*, given that there exist no agreed standards underlying their individual decisions?
3 Is the MRCGP exam a test of competence suitable for certification purposes, given that it was conceived as a test of quality practice?
4 Is there a place for an 'endpoint' assessment which aims to define an objective threshold of performance?

The overall quality of training was addressed through inclusion of formative assessment among the minimal criteria for training practice and hospital posts, in line with the opinion that 'deficiencies in training, if they are only identified at the end of training, are an indictment of the training programme and system' (JCPTGP, 1992). The working party noted that there appeared to be

'a growing mood of determination within general practice to recognise that guarantees on basic entry standards are now necessary as a measure to protect the public and the profession from poor practice, to show teachers and trainers whether training has been successful and to let tax payers see whether their money is being spent wisely' (JCPTGP, 1987).

Fundamentally, there existed no guidance to hospital- and practice-based teachers of general practice trainees on what constituted *satisfactory completion* (the only stated criterion for accrediting each module of vocational training). As a result, refusal of a VTR1 or VTR2 was rare and easily challenged.

A further option was considered, incorporating features of both formative and summative assessment, namely continuing assessment. This would mean that each contributory post in the trainees' progress would be subject to some kind of pass/fail process. Continuous assessment would need to be based on some mutually agreed methodology such as the Manchester Rating Scale.

The emergence of a body of EU legislation provided further ingredients for the debate. From 1990, each member country had to introduce a training package for general practice to facilitate the principles of free movement within Europe and mutual recognition of qualifications. The European Directive (Council Directive 93/16/EEC Title IV), mandatory from 1995, required new legislation – the Vocational Training for General Medical Practice (European Requirements) Regulations 1994. The main consequences were:

1 doctors in general practice (even as assistants or locums) must hold the necessary certificate (or specified exemption)
2 each country must appoint a competent authority to oversee this function
3 the functions of the authority are, among other things, to *supervise* training and issue certificates. The JCPTGP was named by the government as the competent authority for general practice in the United Kingdom in 1995. From that time it was required to extend its role beyond issuing certificates to encompass supervision of training.

A new piece of UK legislation, The Medical (Professional Performance) Act 1995, further strengthened the role of the JCPTGP. Applying to all doctors, it indicated that the government was not satisfied with the overall standards of medical performance and wanted tighter regulation by the GMC, the profession's disciplinary body. One obvious response was to have professionally led control of the gateway to independent practice, coupled with provision for extended training at the expense of 'the system' for those found wanting. Thus, the training system should take responsibility for the casualties of the system.

In summary, a combination of professional and societal unease about the adequacy of the existing certification system, European directives regarding reciprocity and government policy on regulation for the profession all pointed toward a combination of formative assessment and summative assessment to ensure minimum standards of training without sacrificing hallmarks of quality. The MRCGP is clearly not an assessment of minimum standards. Justice demands that trainees should not come through the system and be faced with unemployability without safeguards. Despite misgivings about the resource implications and the immediate unpopularity of the move as expressed by many within the system, the Joint Committee adopted the policy of summative assessment aimed at minimum standards of competence.

Initially a professionally led policy, pending arrangements for financing, training procedures and legislation, it becomes mandatory from 1998. Although a *fait accompli*, it is a further step in the incremental development of general practice standards in line with the evolving primary care-led NHS, and not a rigid unchangeable structure.

The two exams

'Questions have arisen as to whether general practice is now introducing a two-tier assessment process. The answer is yes.' (JCPTGP, 1995)

This has posed practical problems:

- workload for all concerned increased substantially, related to the implementation of the necessary changes
- the RCGP modified the style and timing of its examination, partly to accommodate the incipient summative assessment, while developing its own philosophy and individuality
- course organizers and trainers have had to master a flow of new guidelines and regulations specific to both exams and steer registrars through the multiple options – entry dates, times and venues for the multiplicity of exam sittings and deadlines for submission of contributory work.

The teaching role has been complicated by the need to support registrars through the substantial new effort involved, provide additional support for the production of assessed work and assimilate all of this into the expanding curriculum. Teachers have had to take steps to grasp thoroughly the status quo, access up-to-date information and be vigilant about new developments. Any account of the assessment system in vocational training must therefore be regarded as subject to verification and updating from regional office, RCGP or Joint Committee.

The summative assessment

Aim

To ensure attainment of minimum competence before entering general practice.

Objectives

- To define what is meant by minimum competence.
- To develop a variety of methods for testing those areas of competence which are considered essential.
- To facilitate regions in applying these methods to a nationally agreed and monitored standard.

Content

It was realized from the start that a simple, cheap, reliable test of knowledge, such as the MCQ, would fall short of what is meant by a test of competence. Competence implies a body of knowledge which can be deployed skilfully and appropriately in real situations. Thus, the exam was conceived in four parts.

1 *Knowledge*: tested by MCQ.
2 *Skills*: tested by real consultations recorded on video.
3 *Appropriate performance*: tested by an extensive report by the candidate's trainer.
4 *Audit*: to show that the candidate is capable of carrying out and reporting an autonomous project.

The practicalities of taking this exam are clearly explained by Lindsay *et al.* (1996), but it is important to remember that these may change year by year. The MCQ is offered up to four times per year at the discretion of the regional director. It lasts three hours and consists of 300 true/false questions and extended matching questions.

The audit project emphasizes basic audit method according to a simple protocol. This is marked by three members of the regional panel of assessors selected by the regional director and trained for the task according to nationally approved guidelines.

Projects which fail to meet the criteria are referred to a second line of regional assessors who may in turn refer to a national panel. If they are not satisfied the candidate will be required to resubmit within a specified time. Guidance for redrafting is given, and it should be very unusual for a candidate to fail on this component. The usual problems are excessive complexity or failure to adhere to the given protocol. The audit may be carried out and submitted at any time during the three years of vocational training.

Video component

This must be supplied to the regional office on the standard tape which is provided. It must contain real consultations identified on tape and in an accompanying logbook with the time and date. Both the doctor and patient should be audible and visible except when intimate physical examinations are being carried out. The logbook identifies all the consultations sequentially. The candidate is expected to comment on the consultation performance and may raise issues not apparent on the tape, such as how the process may have been affected by circumstances, improved upon and possible alternative approaches.

It is recommended that registrars start early on preparation for this assessment but they may not submit until the final nine months of training. It is marked by two members of a regional panel of trained assessors. Any unsatisfactory or doubtful submissions are referred to the second line of regional assessors who may, in turn, refer on to national level. Unsatisfactory tapes will be returned for resubmission within a defined time limit.

The experience of a pilot project indicates that the candidates can fail this component through not displaying a reasonable range of consultation skills and by showing unsatisfactory clinical practice. These might have been redressed by appropriate analysis in the logbook which demonstrates insight and active learning. Candidates should therefore be encouraged to review their submissions with their trainer.

The trainer's report

This is a more searching and far-reaching document than that traditionally used. It amounts to more than 30 pages of structured and semi-structured questions and copies may be obtained from the regional office.

Consequences

Successful candidates do not obtain a registrable qualification. The regional director, if satisfied, provides a statement of completion of summative assessment which is submitted along with VTR1 and 2 to the JCPTGP in order to obtain the certificate of prescribed experience. Those who fail the assessment, even after referral and resubmission within the time limit, are unable to carry out general practice in any capacity. A further training period of six to 12 months will be offered.

The system came into force in 1996 without a coherent framework for treating the casualties. If they are, by definition, falling short of minimal competence they are unlikely to be helped simply by returning to hospital posts and trying again later. There is a clear need for specially resourced training practices and skilled trainers willing to provide the further training.

The economic implications of the summative assessment are considerable but not fully clarified. The cost is borne by the regions, not by the candidates and at a time when overall NHS expenditure is a continuing problem this financial burden is a significant resource decision.

The title – *Summative Assessment* – is an unsatisfactory one. It appropriates to a particular context the general concept of summative assessment and implies something definitive about it as a process. It sounds intimidating when it is meant to be minimalist and inclusive, and it conveys little to anyone outside the immediate circle of medical training. This is regrettable as it was originally intended, partly, as a public confidence-building measure. A title such as National Diploma in General Practice might be more appropriate. For the time being its more formal title is the UK Regional Advisers' Assessment (UKRA).

The MRCGP exam

Profile

The general aim is to ensure that College membership implies proficiency in every aspect of general practice. Two historical statements of aim were defined by the College:

- 1971 to test the competence of the ordinary GP in his work
- 1978 the assessment of the knowledge and competences of the GP on completion of vocational training.

The dynamic nature of the MRCGP exam is reflected in this early change of emphasis and its structure which has been evolving continually for more than 30 years – hence this survey of its form must be seen as a snapshot of a changing scene. Up-to-date details should be sought by trainers and course organizers on an annual basis from the Examination Department of the RCGP.

From May 1998, there are four separate modules which can be taken in any order or all at once.

1 *Paper 1* lasting three hours, containing elements of the established MEQ and CRQ sections.
2 *Paper 2* a three-hour, machine-marked paper consisting of the familiar MCQ with elements of the CRQ.
3 *Consultation skills,* an assessment of 15 videotaped consultations.
4 *Oral exam*, two similar unstructured orals lasting 20 minutes each.

Additional requirements cover certification of competence in cardiopulmonary resuscitation (CPR) and child health surveillance (CHS).

The modular format introduces a number of significant departures from the established pattern.

- It can be taken in any order over a three-year period from first application.
- Candidates can take the oral module without pre-condition.
- Modular form has necessitated a shift from peer-referenced to criterion-referenced method.
- Compensating mechanisms have been abandoned and all modules must be passed independently; re-sits are available at an extra fee; failure of any module three times means restarting the whole exam, as does failure to complete within three years.

Profile of Paper 1

There are four types of question:

1 to test the knowledge and interpretation of general practice literature
2 to test the ability to evaluate and interpret written material
3 to examine ability to integrate and apply theoretical knowledge and professional values within the setting of primary care in the UK
4 new question formats may appear which test the application of skills in the context of the changes in primary care.

Notes: three-hour paper; 12 or more questions of equal loading; marked by examiners; where there is supplied material to be evaluated, extra time will be allocated.

Profile of Paper 2

There are two sections which are answered on separate structured proformas and marked separately. These are machine marked, so the technical instructions must be carried out, e.g. fill the appropriate 'lozenge' completely, heavily and in pencil. Some untested questions may be included and this could give rise to marginally different versions of the same paper as these questions are evaluated. There is no negative marking.

- *Section A* up to 400 true–false items
- *Section B* up to 100 items, some in extended matching format, some in single-best-answer format.

In general the paper tests critical appraisal, general medicine and surgery, medical specialties (e.g. eyes, ENT), women's health, child health and service management.

The oral exam

Two consecutive 20-minute orals, each before two examiners. There is no essential difference between the two orals. The practice experience questionnaire has been discontinued. Occasionally there is video-recording or a third party observing the process. This is not to assess the candidates but for purposes relating to assessing or training the examiners. The orals are intended to evaluate decision making and professional values.

Pre-certification

Certificates of competence in CHS and CPR must be supplied when entering the consulting skills module. Expenses involved in undertaking these are not covered by the examination fee. As a rule these are resourced by the training scheme. These certificates are valid for three years.

The consulting skills module

The normal method is by assessment of a video containing 15 consultations. Candidates should be selective about the consultations included in their video for a number of reasons:

- all consultations must be technically adequate for assessment. Basic requirements are that doctor and patient must be audible and visible except during intimate examinations
- the tape should contain a variety of consultations which enable the candidate to demonstrate a wide range of consultation skills
- the finished product is the candidate's clinical 'shop window' and should represent best performance
- informed consent is required before any patient can be recorded on video and a signed consent form must accompany each consultation.

The workbook is of great importance since it enables the candidate to comment on the content and background of the consultations, to supply additional information not readily visible and to show insight by critically appraising his own work. The tape should show the time and date of each consultation corresponding to the account in the workbook.

Since this is the main assessed piece of course work, the video should be prepared in close co-operation with the trainer and not finally submitted without being reviewed to screen for obvious errors of omission or commission. There is an alternative procedure available to those who have very great difficulty in producing a video. On special application such candidates may be allowed to undertake a simulated surgery. These take place twice yearly in London.

Membership by Assessment of Performance

An alternative path to Membership is being devised by the RCGP. Aimed at established principals, it is modelled on the existing Fellowship by Assessment. This recognizes the exclusive nature of formal examinations and promises to be more congruent with the principles of adult learning. It will assess evidence of quality, performance and competence within the candidate's own practice context.

How the MRCGP is marked

All components are marked according to detailed schedules by more than one independent examiner. For example, papers are double marked and after orals all four examiners meet and decide together which of the three standard categories the individual has achieved. Details of mark will not be notified but the result of each module will be reported to the candidate as a fail, pass or pass with merit.

To pass the overall exam it is necessary to pass all four modules. Pass with merit in two of the four results in an overall merit pass. Pass with merit in three or four modules results in distinction. Merit grade in any module will be awarded to approximately 25% of the candidates taking that module.

Strenuous efforts have always been made to ensure fairness in marking. The structure of the exam reflects the wish to test competence and employs a variety of approaches to address the balance between validity and reliability and subjects each aspect to searching statistical analysis. Indeed, the MRCGP has, from the start, been a pathfinder for the entire system of medical education. It has greatly influenced the other specialist colleges and the medical schools' approach to assessment. It continues to refine its methods (some might call them instruments of torture) and explore new approaches.

The course organizer's perspective

Course organizers have traditionally been ambivalent about all summative assessment. This stems from:

1 a lack of statutory responsibility for certification – VTR1 and VTR2 are issued by trainers and hospital consultants respectively; course organizers have no power to select or exclude candidates. This powerless state results in identification with the learners and being a supportive ally to the trainers
2 a growing appreciation that day-release time is limited and should be used for what groups do best – group work aimed at personal and professional growth. This is facilitated by the open and non-threatening position of the course organizer

3 a conviction that assessment, intrinsic to any conscious educational process, should be formative and educative, in line with adult-to-adult relationships espoused by many educationalists – the education *v* training debate.

Thus, in 1988 the ACO rejected the MRCGP as the endpoint of training, expressing the view that this also threatened to be the point at which learning ended. Some of these reservations have been addressed by subsequent developments:

1 in neither exam have course organizers been forced to take a substantial role
2 there has been growth in standards of practice in the CME area which address the inherent problems of continuing learning
3 decisions about the desirability of summative assessment have been taken out of the profession's hands by legislation from both the UK government and the European Union
4 formative assessment has been enshrined among the basic requirements of both hospital and practice training.

The user-friendly role of the course organizer has survived relatively unscathed the turbulent years of the early 1990s. However, we cannot easily escape the perception by others, notably trainers and registrars, that the day-release course will provide some element of classroom teaching which will contribute substantially towards exam success. We cannot fully escape the feeling that 'failure' by a registrar is, to some extent, our failure too.

We ourselves are subject to unsophisticated forms of assessment. Whereas it is difficult to gauge the extent to which our groups contribute to increased 'wholeness and maturity' of the trainees, it is easy to ask 'why did X% of your group fail the exams?', accompanied by telling comparisons with the neighbouring schemes. Thus, in 1993 the ACO reluctantly accepted the logic of the arguments expressed by the JCPTGP. Despite misgivings about the political climate out of which they emerged and positions adopted in relation to educational principles, it merely advised its members to avoid personal involvement in the summative assessment of trainees from their own group. In general, opposition to summative assessment and its philosophy has collapsed.

The continuing debates are educative for all. The main regrets of course organizers relate to:

• the increased level of stress experienced by the majority of their registrars who elect to undertake both examinations at the end of the course
• the competing demands on the day-release course
• the moral imperative to contribute towards the overall exam preparation tasks which are high on the priority list of both registrars and trainers.

UKRA addresses some prior anomalies. Formerly, the JCPTGP was responsible for standards of training and regional advisers for the provision of a satisfactory training programme, but neither had any direct control over endpoint assessment. The college exam tended to fulfil this function progressively, without substantial challenge and without responsibility for the training process or resource implications. It was an external form of summative assessment relating to neither the teachers nor the governing body of vocational training.

UKRA now represents the philosophy and the standard setting role of the Joint Committee which represents the stakeholders (the academic and service wings of the profession) and is constituted as the Responsible Authority embodied by domestic and European legislation. Under its guidance and examining body is the UK Conference of Regional Advisers. The UKRA exam is implemented by the regional director, who is also responsible for the total implementation and resourcing of vocational training.

This brings about a separation between certification for practice, with its attendant protection of the interests of the public and profession, and the college exam, freeing the latter to be the badge of lifelong membership of a learned body whose interests are wholly educational. This may impinge on the numbers electing for college membership. A new challenge is therefore presented to the College and its exam system since the UKRA exam becomes the certification endpoint. The two most likely options are:

1 revert to its original vision of being an elective test of young principals as they become established in their career
2 continue to participate in a two-tier system of endpoint assessment of training with, perhaps, gradual convergence between the two systems.

Looking forward

Vocational training is undergoing changes which will have a bearing on the timing and structure of the assessment tasks. In 1997 the ACO recommended that all three years of VT should be general practice based (ACO, 1997). More conservatively, the Calman Report (1995) recommended that the practice based period of training should expand from the minimum of 12 months to at least 18 months, if necessary at the expense of the hospital-based components. This will expand the period of training specific to general practice, reducing the current level of pressure in the training practice and day-release course. Trainees will probably experience more than one training practice with a separate VTR1 from each.

Recent moves by the JCPTGP, specialty Royal Colleges and SCOPME are geared towards improving the experience of hospital-based training (see Part 4). There is more emphasis on teaching based on agreed curriculum aims and more systematic continuing assessment, including periodic appraisal of SHOs before the VTR2 certificates are signed.

This begins to resemble a credit accumulation transfer system (CATS) whereby trainees collect separate credits from a variety of learning situations. It is possible to envisage an expansion of the range of pre-certifications, over and above the two currently required for the MRCGP, to encompass other, wider skills or learning modules taken at various times during training. A possible candidate for this could be in the area of IT skills.

These trends constitute the basis of portfolio-based learning, comprising formative assessment, transferable credits, continuous assessment with summative elements in-built and, if still necessary, some form of endpoint assessment which need not necessarily take examination form.

Assuming the two-tier exam system survives there is a further conceivable division of labour. The Merrison Report of 1976 recommended the adoption of two tiers of training (for all specialties) – basic professional training (BPT) of three years and higher professional training (HPT) for two years. In general practice only the first level has been achieved and the RCGP is actively exploring the implications of five-year training and the introduction of HPT programmes. Clearly the UKRA exam could serve as the endpoint of basic training. The trainee might enter clinical practice while still undertaking higher training, with MRCGP as the endpoint and definitive specialist qualification. At present the College does not favour this role for its membership exam.

The RCGP Fellowship by Assessment process would then complete the ladder of quality and competence, providing a clear, if arduous, pathway of career development which general practice has historically lacked. The resource implications are formidable and the effects on the world of general practice difficult to foresee but these are issues that the College working party on HPT is addressing.

It may be professionally unacceptable to further lengthen the path to definitive practice which could threaten the unity and essential egalitarianism of general practice. It would alter the GP's terms of service by opening up the prospect of two-tier practice – those with HPT and MRCGP being the principals (essentially specialists in family practice) with a second level composed of assistants and locums who do not get beyond BPT and UKRA certification. It could all become a bureaucratic, ivory tower building, divisive and expensive nightmare. The protection against such a disastrous scenario remains, as always, the twin perspectives of the GP teacher – developments in professional training should always seek to be patient centred and learner sensitive.

Examination preparation

To what extent should you take into account the requirements of the examinations as you plan your curriculum? In deciding this you should consider the views of the trainees, trainers and regional director, recognizing that:

- there is a demand for exams by trainees, the profession and society
- the UKRA is mandatory
- there is merit in having a motivating goal at the end of training
- much of what vocational training offers is tested in the exams.

If you decide that this is important there are several methods to consider. Some are routine elements of day-release teaching and assessment.

1 Past test papers: the MEQ is particularly versatile and not just for examination preparation. It is useful for finding weak spots in clinical knowledge. Past papers of the MRCGP are jealously guarded, but there are useful books of tests with model answers. The format of the exam is changing at such a rate that past papers are of limited value.
2 Organizing pre-certification procedures. Cardiopulmonary resuscitation is good day-release course fare. Certifying competence in child health surveillance is normally the province of the trainer.
3 The journal reading syndicate is a universal feature of vocational training. The evidence-based and critical reading emphases are important provided they do not paradoxically limit the scope of the trainees' reading.
4 The mock exam, a full-scale replica of papers and orals, is laborious but educative for all concerned.
5 'Exam-cram' courses are run by some regions and the RCGP. They relieve pressure on the day-release course but are expensive.
6 All course organizers should be able to provide information and respond to trainees' questions about the examinations. Regulations change. The sources of information are, for the UKRA, the Regional Office and for the MRCGP, the Examination Department of the Royal College of General Practitioners.

Scenario: Assessment

Meeke: *This assessment business is getting out of hand, I hate it.*
Best: *Good, I was just about to pour myself a drink and ask you what you wanted to talk about next. I think we could both do with one – it's a weighty topic. White or red?*
Meeke: *Red please. I don't know where to start!*
Best: *It seems to me you have feelings on the matter. Let's start there.*
Meeke: *I hate it when you say that. Now I know how the trainees feel when I do it to them. I want to talk about the mess things are getting into at the course and you want me to talk about my feelings.*
Best: *We will talk about assessment, after you've told me how much you hate it.*

Meeke: *I hate it because I don't know where I'm at with it. OK, feelings...disorientated, all at sea, overloaded, drowning in paper. How's that for a start?*

Best: *Not bad for a golfer. Maybe you've hit rock bottom, finding it's not all plain sailing. But enough of the maritime images...where has this come from?*

Meeke: *I've just been at a regional meeting about assessment. Hours of boring discussion about changes in the MRCGP and this summative assessment examination. Then we had some stuff about validity, reliability, discrimination, criterion-referenced and peer-referenced standards, all sorts of technical stuff. Then there were entry dates for this, submission dates for that, pre-certification for the other, three or four different times in the year for each of the bits of both examinations. If it's upsetting me I hate to think what the trainees will make of it. Then there were regulations about the audits, the length and quality of the videos needed for each examination.*

Best: *Listening to you makes me feel not so bad about retirement. Let's step back a bit and think about what assessment is for rather than the mechanics of it.*

Meeke: *I'm not finished hating yet. I think I was led up the garden path when I took on this job. All the ACO stuff I read before I started was about the virtues of formative assessment – working with the trainees to explore for gaps in their knowledge and how to remedy them; how every aspect of the day-release course should tell us something about their progress in terms of knowledge, skills and attitudes. Then I went on the small group course and was persuaded that the course is really about sensitivity training and personal growth work. They would come out more mature, rounded doctors who could listen to their patients and this would come through in their examination performance. Now we have a steeple-chase with fences and water-jumps to face as well. I'm thinking about getting out.*

Best: *What's stopping you?*

Meeke: *I can't walk away from my group just because I'm feeling fed up, can I? No. I'll have to see it through to the end of the year. Then I'm out.*

Best: *Did you ever hear of mid-term blues? It's a bit like seasonal affective disorder, feeling sad because all you see is the clouds when what you need is some light. It's not an unusual feeling half way through the year – lots of work has been put in, the programme is full of loose ends, the trainees are beginning to feel restless because they can see the time running out and examinations looming and there is the feeling that it won't all come together in the end. Are you picking up pressure from the group?*

Meeke: *I suppose I am. A few months ago they were really getting into things like how to tackle psychosocial problems at the surgery, what to do about addiction, they even wanted to try a Balint group. Now all they want is stuff about the evidence for interval breast cancers and to collect journal references like magpies. Anything that's not going to get them through the critical reading paper seems to them like a waste of time – they want more practice test papers, more journal clubs, more clinical lectures. I feel they are driving me rather than me educating them. Sorry, I meant facilitating them.*

Best: *I think you may still have a romantic view of education. Was that a Freudian slip you just made? Maybe there is a tug of war going on within you. You want them to pass the examinations and get their certificate and get into good practices – right? You also want them to make discoveries about themselves and how they develop their intuitions, be patient-centred problem-solvers, self-directed learners, sensitive but efficient managers of teams and all these wonderful vision statements. Good. What do they want?*

Meeke: *I suppose I should ask them.*

Best: *What is their behaviour telling you?*

Meeke: *They want to pass the examinations and get good practices and they want me to help them do it.*

Best: *So what's the problem? Why not give them what they want?*

Meeke: *Because I'm afraid that what they want isn't good enough. I know for a fact that some of them haven't read a book so far this year and I'm not talking about the Oxford Textbook. They haven't read Balint nor Neighbour nor Pendleton nor the College book nor...*

Best: *...and I bet they don't listen to Radio 4, play the piano or read Kafka! They're busy and they've a lot on their plate. Those other things will come – they will be GPs for a long time.*

Meeke: *Hey, whose side are you on? It was you who fed me a lot of stuff about discovering the inner self, to believe in something called wisdom or professionalism, to want to get to the roots of people's problems. My real fear is that the examination fetish is pushing all that out of sight. We have often heard that examination systems guarantee that people will stop learning when the examination is over – the 'never again' syndrome. I tell you, not one of them will want to critically appraise a paper again after May this year.*

Best: *Well, tell me, how often have you critically appraised a paper since you became a GP? Don't you see that once you learn the skill of critical reading you'll never again read a journal the same way. It works its way into critical thinking, and that is likely to stick. And if it doesn't stick straight away give them a year or two in practice and they'll be coming up with questions that need answers – moral dilemmas, decisions about practice policies, use of resources, guidelines – that sort of thing. At least they'll know where the library is which is more than can be said for a lot of wise old men I know who never had the benefit of an action-packed trainee year.*

Meeke: *That's quite a sermon. Do you think I'm wrong about all this?*

Best: *Not at all. What has stirred us both up is our old friend cognitive dissonance – the tension between what is and what should be. That's what makes us think and act. Now, I bet the Regional Adviser didn't say you could stop formative assessment just because a whole extra load of summative assessment has dropped from on high.*

Meeke: *That's right, we're expected to do both; keep records of progress, chat to the trainees about their individual weak points and get them through the exams.*

Best: *This reminds me of the famous question about an American President: 'Can he walk and chew gum at the same time?' Time to talk about the 'how to' of all this. What comes to mind? Keep it simple, now.*

Meeke: *Well, I suppose I could prepare an information sheet for them summarizing the examination requirements. Regional office could do most of that for me.*
  – Turn the groupwork slots into a problem-based approach so that they find out what the literature says about a few main clinical areas and explore the controversies
  – Give them a few examination papers to practise on and make a note of how they do
  – Use their examination videos to touch on consultation issues
  – Get them to bring in their audit projects, discuss what that contributes to the practice, maybe even put up a small prize for the best. How am I doing?

Best: *Great. And what about giving them time to talk about their feelings on assessment? How's the wine, by the way.*

Meeke: *We've been so busy talking I've hardly noticed, sorry. It's got a good nose, full-bodied, very fruity – must be French.*

Best: *Wrong, it's Chilean, but you've just done some assessment. You got the main points. Anyone who can correctly assess something as abstract as taste and smell shouldn't have any bother assessing the finer points of training for general practice. Assess some more of this and enjoy it this time.*

8

Curriculum development

'Students graduate – overwhelmed with learning but in urgent need of worldly understanding.' (Samuel, 1990a)

Introduction

Curricula evolve. Few people have the opportunity to construct a complete new course from first principles. Even if one had such an opportunity it would not work. Curriculum development is not a paper exercise. As the term implies it is a process of defining goals, then planning, implementing, reviewing and refining them. In course organizing, as in management or audit, many activities which appear at first sight to be linear turn out to be cyclical.

The curriculum development cycle is normally applied to aspects of the course in turn rather than the whole course at once. It is difficult to work effectively in a situation where everything is in flux. If there are no fixed points there is a risk of disorientation.

This chapter does not aim to produce a core curriculum or a master copy of a programme for the day-release course, but to present the elements of curriculum planning and development from which practical guidelines may be deduced.

The curriculum: what is it?

Curriculum is a peculiar animal. Its functional life depends on its integrity, how it relates to the other main educational functions. It needs:

- a lively understanding of the educational philosophy (the formulation of beliefs and values) which underlie the course

- the resources which are available in the educational setting. In a shrinking economy is it 'the tail that wags the dog'?
- four legs of more or less equal strength: aims (the goals of training), methods (the 'how' of teaching), assessment (the feedback loops which measure how aims are being achieved, suggest corrective action and identify new learning tasks) and programming (the organization of educational elements which make up the course).

This animal is versatile, it experiences growth, may be influenced by other members of the same species (interdisciplinary learning) and may even function quite well in the face of handicap (it is unusual for an animal to be in perfect health all the time). As a course organizer are you the creator, the jockey or the vet?

Definitions

Rogers (1986) suggested three definitions of curriculum.

1 Curriculum = Method + Content.
2 A body of knowledge to which the learner must be exposed.
3 All the planned experiences to which the learner may be exposed in order to achieve the learning goals.

To these I would add a 'quasi-definition':

4 The purpose of a curriculum is to facilitate assessment. (Is there a tendency to write the curriculum when it seems we are likely to be inspected?)

However debatable the last definition, it is clear that in educational systems which relate to summative assessment, the *curriculum* closely resembles the *syllabus* for the terminal examinations. This sort of curriculum is the teacher's guide for covering the course set by the examiners. It suggests lists of contents, aims and objectives, well worked out with regard to knowledge of the subject matter. It focuses attention on the teacher teaching. It is teacher centred and content oriented.

Centredness and orientation in the curriculum

'*I have to ask on what the curriculum is based if it is not centred on the students.*' (Cross, 1975)

There is evidence that the different forms of assessment affect not just what is learned, but how the learning happens (*see* Chapter 6). To allow the curriculum to become learner centred, the emphasis should shift from terminal or summative assessment to the assessment of interim objectives and the identification of learning needs (formative assessment). The purpose of a learner-centred curriculum is to make learning as effective as possible, taking into account individual learning styles, life situations and goals. The traditional exam-oriented syllabus produces a view of the curriculum which is content centred, and this is reflected in the increasing exam orientation of vocational training. It produces a checklist approach and influences the selection of teaching methods, favouring the didactic approach and a convergent cognitive style. In the educational setting of the day-release course, where the end-product is not clearly definable and the participants are autonomous adults, a conflict of values results. Broader educational aims lend themselves better to formative assessment and to learning processes which emphasize interaction, reflection and exploration. This requires process orientation rather than content orientation.

Some thoughts on learner – and teacher – centredness

An educational setting which is totally learner centred may be a recipe for chaos, especially if it is totally process oriented. Learner-centredness is not learner domination.

A teacher-centred, content-oriented curriculum is a prescription for repression of ideas and is unconducive to freeing learners to grow.

As course organizers we have a duty to take responsibility for the course. If we relinquish being teacher centred we still cannot devolve our responsibilities to the trainees unless we adopt an extreme view of trainee-centredness. Rogers (1986) suggested that all teachers can locate themselves on a grid based on two orthogonal scales as shown in Figure 8.1.

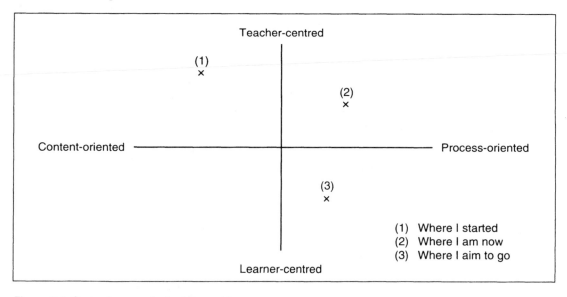

Figure 8.1 Centredness and orientation grid.

Exercise 12

(a) Where are you located on the centredness/orientation grid? In which direction would you like your grid reference to shift, and why?

(b) Any shift implies that the teacher is learning through the teaching process. Who is teaching whom? What is the teacher learning?

As with any distribution of behaviour or attitude, a position at the periphery requires some explanation, especially if it is consistently maintained across the range of different curriculum areas and activities, or does not change with time and experience.

Implications of learner-centredness/process orientation

1 The curriculum will be based on methods which are interactive and inclusive and will emphasize peer learning.
2 Active learning will be fostered through participation in group-learning tasks and action learning.
3 The needs of the individual will be addressed through formative assessment and encouragement to participate in affective learning opportunities within the group, with feedback.
4 The year's activities will focus on themes rather than subjects, so that participants can formulate principles rather than learn facts.
5 Learning tasks for the year will emphasize the development of skills which will enhance autonomous practice, especially in such areas as information processing, communication and management.
6 Expert input to the course will be employed to supplement the trainees' self-learning activities. The course organizer will brief resource persons in advance about the learning needs of the group.
7 The trainee group will be helped to participate in all aspects of the learning process, including assessment and curriculum planning.

The course curriculum: where does it come from?

The day-release course curriculum is a multi-layered structure. At the base is the theoretical layer – the implications of the decision about centredness and orientation.

The second layer consists of the strategic planning of the course, with its priorities and methods. The top layer is the most tangible, comprising curriculum features and activities which make up the programme. Every course organizer has a curriculum, and it is worth asking whether yours came about by:

- *Inheritance.* Most new course organizers inherit much that is valuable from their predecessor
- *Prescription.* No course is autonomous. Each region has an educational strategy and a mini-culture developed over the years. You fit into this somehow and your ideas tend to develop within this framework
- *Prefabrication.* Curriculum features are borrowed from other people, even from other disciplines
- *Creation.* Do you try to make new GPs in your own image or based on your own learning needs?
- *Democracy.* This only works if the trainees know what they want. Usually, however, they don't know what they don't know, so you are tempted to write the term timetable yourself
- *Pragmatism.* You look at MRCGP papers and decide how best to get the trainees through.

Since your course has a pre-existing curriculum, your initial tasks are to grasp its meaning and structure, to implement and experiment with it. You should aim to develop the curriculum rather than to create the perfect course from scratch. This is frequently a team activity, undertaken in conjunction with fellow course organizers within the local scheme or at the regional course organizers' workshops. The priorities are to discern the underlying educational values, and examine each of the programme building-blocks continually and critically, to assess and revise them, trying to innovate where possible. There is no general agreement yet about what constitutes the core curriculum of vocational training for general practice. In any case much of it is, at present, in the hands of hospital- and practice-based teachers. This is why it is important to have good lines of communication with local consultants and trainers' workshop. Some help may be got from the recently defined core activities of the GP (GMSC, 1996), the General Medical Council list of attributes essential for any doctor (GMC, 1987) and the Joint Committee's formulation of the attributes of the GP (JCPTGP, 1997). Significantly, the Joint Committee regards the attainment of these attributes as the curriculum aim of vocational training.

Very full and thoughtful accounts of the concepts which underlie vocational training, with special reference to the training practice, appear in Samuel (1990a), the Oxford Region report on priorities (RCGP, 1988) and the new Manchester Rating Scales (RCGP, 1989). These might be critically examined by each course organizer in conjunction with the trainers' workshop as an aid to curriculum planning, so that a 'locally owned' programme can take into account the division of labour between the hospital component, the practice year and the day-release course. Curriculum issues relating to the hospital component are considered in Tait (1987), a Royal College of Physicians report (RCP, 1997) and the RCGP series of agreed learning objectives for SHOs published in 1993 (*see* Part 4).

Everyone will want a say in your curriculum (not just the regional directors, trainers and trainees whose contributions are quite legitimate):

- various hospital specialist groups ('GPs need to know more about orthopaedics, genetic counselling' etc.)
- pressure groups ('young GPs are taught nothing about the aftermath of nuclear war, domestic violence' etc.)
- commercial interests who want to sell you their latest educational package (and 'have a wee word' with the trainees at the same time).

With limited time and resources you cannot meet everyone's demands. You need to become highly selective concerning the content of the day-release course.

Three useful principles were formulated at the 1985 ACO Conference (Seiler, 1986).

1 The release course should attempt to do what cannot be done elsewhere.
2 The group should concentrate on doing what the group does best.
3 The whole group should be involved in setting out the programme for the term.

Each region has a 'mission statement' of educational aims for the scheme, which should be read carefully when formulating curriculum aims. Weston (1986) provided one such statement of principles:

Aim
to assist participants to improve their emotional and intellectual understanding of all aspects of whole-person medicine and how to practise it.

Objectives
to create a peer-learning community where emotional and intellectual learning can occur; to provide educational activities not available elsewhere; and to produce a curriculum based on the agreed needs of participants.

The curriculum: what goes in?

Samuel (1990b) suggested that the content of the curriculum includes three main elements: facts, concepts and values. These are not separate commodities but elements which may be present in any one activity. Even the most conventional lecture may encompass all three.

Facts

The factual element in the day-release curriculum is important but incidental, being more central to hospital and practice components. '*If we accept that most clinical skills in general practice are currently best taught in training practices or hospital outpatients and that factual knowledge can be generally learned from books, then one of the principal aims of the day-release course is in the area of sensitivity training for doctors'* (Editorial, 1986).

Factual learning is most important when there is new material, or there are inter-disciplinary topics which need special resourcing, or in response to an identified knowledge gap in the group. Such situations are identified by the course organizer in conjunction with the trainees and trainers' workshop.

It is perhaps more useful to talk about knowledge: a store of facts organized in relation to previous experience which can be applied actively to new situations. The trainees' knowledge is not a consequence of the day-release course but the soil out of which the course grows. This soil needs working over and enriching. This will be considered later in relation to the clinical content of the day-release course. *'Knowledge is information that works'* (Neighbour, 1996).

Concepts

'In order to develop the curriculum, the concepts on which our daily work is based need to be identified and defined.' (Samuel, 1990b)

According to Samuel, the concepts include:

- self-responsibility (the ability to hold and express opinions, to change and to initiate change)
- commitment to a lifetime of professional study
- respect for the patient's autonomy
- the ability to respond with empathy to patients who need support (this could be expanded to include behaviour towards staff, colleagues and family).

In addition to Samuel's list, I would emphasize a further category: methodology. This relates to how we acquire and service the intellectual tools of our trade, and how we evaluate, apply, store and retrieve knowledge. It is clearly exemplified in the critical reading parts of the MRCGP exam and would include information processing, for those who feel they are drowning in paper.

Values

There is no such thing as a value-free practice of medicine. We should, therefore, be helping the trainees to make personal discoveries about beliefs (their own and other people's), foster values that are appropriate, and encourage them to practise making and reviewing sound value judgements. In this way they develop their own sense of ethical values, along with a critical faculty for identifying their own and other people's ethical assumptions. Values are seldom directly explored by a curriculum. They are more often approached in an opportunistic fashion with an emphasis on experiential or action learning through activities such as group work (especially Balint work), projects, debates and problem case analysis. The relative absence of teaching about ethics and values at the earlier stages of professional development means that there may be a need for remedial teaching in this area.

EXAMPLE

Maureen presents a case: *A middle-aged man presents with a 'bad back'. Through repeated consultations his problem defies all attempts to relieve it, though he never appears to be in pain. After some exploration he discloses that his wife has advanced multiple sclerosis, but he does not want to talk about her. There is a hint about an insurance claim pending. He needs further sickness certification. Maureen feels frustrated at the lack of progress with the back problem; she feels manipulated, but also sympathetic on account of his wife.*
   Can the group help her explore the issues?

Approaches to specific learning tasks

The use of checklists

'What is the point of completing the syllabus if the learner does not really learn?... It is better to focus on a sample of the content and help the learners to do the rest for themselves...to create a desire to pursue an acquaintance with methods of continual learning.' (Rogers, 1986)

Checklists have been a feature of vocational training for many years, especially in the training practice, as a tool for curriculum planning and self-assessment. From the checklist, topics can be shortlisted and educational strategies devised around each for inclusion in the programme. Checklists can be helpful so long as the course organizer is selective. *One should not attempt to create a comprehensive and exhaustive list of items covering knowledge, skills and attitudes in general practice.*

Instructional objectives

'Aims are things you can't measure. Objectives are things you can measure.' (Gronlund, 1978)

General instructional outcome: *uses critical thinking skills in reading.*

Specific outcomes: *the learner*

- distinguishes between facts and opinions
- distinguishes between facts and inferences
- identifies cause and effect relations
- identifies errors in reasoning
- distinguishes between relevant and irrelevant argument
- distinguishes between warranted and unwarranted generalizations
- formulates valid conclusions from written material
- specifies assumptions needed to make conclusions true

Figure 8.2 Teaching/learning exercise on critical reading (Gronlund, 1978).

The behaviourist approach to education suggests that the course content can be broken down into a finite, manageable number of *general instructional objectives.*

1 Each general instructional objective is stated in terms of one general learning outcome (behaviour).
2 Each general learning outcome gives rise to an array of specific learning outcomes.
3 These specific learning outcomes constitute a sample of behaviours sufficient to indicate the attainment of the objective.
4 The list of specific outcomes should be comprehensive enough to clarify the instructional content and short enough to be manageable and useful.
5 The exercise should be learner centred, i.e. centred on what the learner learns rather than on what the teacher teaches and it should focus on learning outcomes rather than process.

An example of instructional objectives for a learner-centred exercise is shown in Figure 8.2.

The outcomes are observable behaviours, not abstract processes. This method is applicable to simple educational tasks, and may even further the learning of complex specific tasks like critical reading (when they are definable). Problems arise in the use of these methods when the desired behavioural outcomes are undefined, subtle or wide-ranging. Consequently, planning by objectives has not been generally successful or widely adopted in UK general practice training (Samuel, 1990a) but some successful rating scales adopt this format.

The behavioural approach may be useful in the planning of specific learning exercises such as:

- a session about setting up mini-clinics at the surgery

- a seminar on asthma management
- a module on problem drinking.

This approach can help you focus more clearly on content, methods and appropriate assessment procedures. It is favoured by educators in the USA where training curricula for family medicine programmes consist of immensely detailed lists of specific competences with respective assessment criteria and teaching hours. The British tradition is more interested in defining aims and process.

The trainers' workshop and the curriculum

The contribution of the trainers' workshop to the process of formulating the day-release course curriculum has already been referred to. Its central task in this respect is to identify those learning areas and tasks which are more appropriately undertaken in a group setting or which depend on the specific resources available at the postgraduate centre. Some overlap is unavoidable and may be beneficial when the complementary nature of the practice and day-release course settings is being deliberately exploited, for example in modular work and action learning.

Day-release course activities frequently reveal individual learning needs. These can be discussed with the trainee and appropriately highlighted for remedial treatment with the trainer. The trainers' workshop may be encouraged to meet specific learning needs of trainees, e.g. with practice exchanges. Trainers should take part in the day-release course as resource persons in turn.

Clinical medicine in the day-release course

The field is so huge that it is best to start out with generalities rather than specifics. The focus may therefore be on three main areas.

1 *Principles of method.* Educational approaches to clinical topics should emphasize the distinctive methodology of general practice, based on core concepts such as:
   - communication and consultation
   - prevention and health education
   - prescribing principles
   - family dynamics
   - interdisciplinary teamwork.
2 *General management plans,* emphasizing transferable knowledge and skills, can include topics such as:
   - chronic disease
   - terminal care

- addiction
- behaviour disorders
- the ill child
- 'medicine after midnight'
- sexually transmitted diseases.

Clearly the production of guidelines in these areas entails a good deal of detailed discussion of clinical and structural issues.

3 *Target diseases.* Some specific clinical conditions are of such significance that they merit consideration in some detail. Examples of suitable topics include:

- coronary artery disease
- obstructive airways disease
- peptic ulcer and reflux syndrome
- anxiety and depression
- AIDS.

Whilst practical clinical skills are not primarily the concern of the course organizer, it may be necessary to co-ordinate practical instruction on behalf of the trainers, who may not have the necessary resources. These include cardiopulmonary resuscitation, joint injection and other minor surgery skills.

A new curriculum?

'The evolving scope of the job description of the GP in the UK, as primary physician, commissioner of care, health promoter and gatekeeper for hospital and community resources, generates educational challenges for vocational training.' (McEvoy, 1995)

Developments in NHS practice in the 1990s, embodied in the 1990 GP contract and the purchaser–provider split, have altered the balance of content in the curriculum of the day-release course. The prevalent emphasis on personal development is giving way to an appreciation of management skills (*see* Chapter 14). Further pressures on the learning agenda arise from the introduction of summative assessment in 1996, well in advance of any expansion of practice-based learning time.

Major factors which also need to be assimilated include the increasing emphasis on evidence-based practice, the concern about ethical awareness (especially in relation to family and reproductive issues), medical economics (resource utilization and rationing of care) and information technology.

The curriculum for the year 2000 looks radically different from that of the 1980s. Reforms in the balance between hospital- and practice-based learning will profoundly affect the scope and content of day-release training. There will be more disposable time, but that will be accompanied by more decisions about what to include and how to integrate, sequence and programme learning. The crisis in recruitment is resulting in smaller training schemes, fallow training practices (and fallow course organizers) and increasing numbers of medical graduates from other EU countries. These come from very different medical systems and learning cultures and may present special needs. Plans are at an advanced stage for innovative higher professional training, being piloted in the form of vocationally trained associates, a creative consequence of the Tomlinson Report and the formation of the London Incentive Zone Educational Initiative (LIZEI) (Salmon and Savage, 1997). This will take on and develop some aspects of the present basic training.

New learning approaches should be developed to meet these curriculum challenges. One which merits close scrutiny is problem-based learning (PBL). It is not much in evidence in postgraduate medical education outside the Netherlands and Norway. However, it is rapidly making an impact on undergraduate curricula and, before long, it will be a learning approach familiar to new generations of trainees. For this reason, if for no other, it is something that course organizers ought to know about.

Problem-based learning

'PBL is an important means towards developing and maintaining creatively and critically reasoning practitioners who are well equipped to pursue self-directed learning throughout their professional life.' (Engel, 1992)

Problem-based learning is a dialectical method of education which embraces a 'bottom-up' rather than the traditional 'top-down' approach. In PBL the desired learning objectives are identified, and a process constructed to encompass these with a minimum of unnecessary effort. This is done through posing problem scenarios related to real experience. It is group based and the group task is to discuss and research the ramifications of each question, commission any specialized assistance required to further the process and to reflect on what has been learned. The PBL emphasis is on a sequence of wide-ranging but specific learning aims, active learning and freedom to identify and choose relevant methods and objectives. By the end of the course the ramifications of the individual exercises should interlock to create an adequate knowledge base. In the process the learner acquires and develops a grasp of methodology, perhaps at some expense in comprehensiveness of knowledge. This contrasts with the traditional curriculum concept of learning the rudiments of basic sciences and contributing disciplines in the hope that they will provide a comprehensive repertoire of knowledge, assuming that good teaching and good memory will achieve good outcomes.

Questions arise concerning the outcome of either system in terms of professional competence. Studies show that PBL promotes lasting skills in accessing information, assessing evidence and self-directed learning. Graduates from either type of course converge in clinical knowledge and ability shortly after graduating (Ferrier, 1990; Woodward, 1989). There is reason to believe that PBL graduates have enhanced ability to transfer concepts to new problems and they retain the specific skills which equip them for continuing learning. Significantly, the process is shown to be enjoyable and satisfying for learners and teachers (Bligh, 1995) while fostering the preferred deep approach to learning (Newble and Clarke, 1986).

The impact of PBL has been at undergraduate level. A handful of new medical schools were founded in the 1960s and 1970s based entirely on the PBL approach, notably McMaster (Canada), Newcastle (Australia) and Maastricht (Netherlands), to name but a few of the more eminent ones. These institutions have had a disproportionate influence on undergraduate medical education, as well as contributing at graduate level the philosophy of evidence-based practice. Now many UK medical schools are radically reforming their curricula along PBL lines.

In view of the vast literature establishing the effectiveness of PBL for students in medicine and allied professions and the growing conviction among academics that this is the future for medical schools, why is it not applied to general, higher or continuing professional training? One might speculate that it is difficult to cross over from one learning tradition to another. Teachers coming from the 'old school' may be resistant to reorienting their teaching styles. PBL is also more time and labour intensive than mass instructional techniques such as the lecture/seminar. This is because it is based on small group learning. It therefore requires from the teachers skills in leading small groups and a high degree of responsive flexibility to address the specific learning needs identified by the group as it processes each problem. The process of PBL is as follows:

- *Creating the curriculum.* The curriculum is designed like a grid or a section through a layer cake. The core curriculum is reduced to a manageable number of learning aims. An underlying layer consists of generic concepts which ought to be covered. In the process of exploring each of the core aims enough of these objectives should be covered to constitute a reasonable breadth of curriculum. The next layer down is a plan of the resources which the group might need to consult or employ – the contribution of various specialists, 'skills lab' sessions, library facilities and fieldwork. Then at the bottom there is the assessment layer. Appropriate assessments are planned for each exercise. Finally, the icing is applied – the limited list of problems through which the group will enter into the process, exploring the layers underneath. Each aim is formulated as a reality-based problem, usually in the form of a carefully constructed open question such as: *'Mrs Roberts, aged 60, consults you saying that, although she read in a newspaper that HRT causes cancer, she heard that it would help her osteoporosis'.*
- *The tutorial.* The typical group session lasts two to three hours. Members elect a chairman and recorder and begin by brainstorming the question. They then proceed to problem posing, identifying the main thrusts of inquiry. This is followed by

task setting – each member decides what aspects of the scenario he will research in preparation for the next meeting. *What are the risks of various cancers with/without HRT; effects of HRT on cardiovascular risk; the consequences of osteoporosis; overall cost?*

- *Individual work.* Group members explore the topic in as much breadth and depth as possible – *reading; Internet; discuss with trainer/local expert.*
- *The follow-up tutorial.* The group meets again to discuss the question, their findings and reflect critically on what each has learned. *Outcome: useful; want to explore other issues in women's health.*
- *Next.* This is followed by addressing the next PBL cycle. Unfinished business from the exercise (such as knowledge gaps) can be identified for personal study or, if substantial, set up as a further, elective PBL exercise.
- *The group tutor.* Throughout the tutorials the tutor is present in a non-expert capacity. This can be any member of staff and he might not have any special expertise on the topic. His role is to give advice about approaches, procedure, resources, make sensible suggestions and help sort out difficulties.

The group learns to work together as a collective, to take responsibility for its own learning, to identify and meet its own needs, and to learn the leadership and conflict resolution skills of teamwork.

Clearly this process has evolved in medical schools where there is a full faculty of teachers at the service of the learners and committed to this style of teaching. Of what relevance, then, is PBL to vocational training?

Many day-release courses have functioned, in reality, within the confines of one academic year. The curriculum of GP training is, like the universe, without boundaries and still expanding. The approach must, therefore, be one of sampling rather than covering it. Preparing for a lifetime of working in a multidisciplinary team within a primary care-led NHS means that essential aims must include teamwork, IT use in the service of evidence-based decision making, and laying the foundations for continuing autonomous or practice-based learning.

If achieving this could be combined with learning interpersonal skills, leadership and insight into how knowledge can be deployed for the benefit of the individual patient, then we are talking about a powerful educational approach, closely resembling an ideal specification.

The PBL approach holds out the promise of all of these. In vocational training in the UK we already have in place the network of small learning groups with skilled group leaders. Each learner has a personal tutor and the resources of the training practice with its library, IT capacity and multiprofessional team. Each NHS district has resources which include primary and secondary care specialists, and fieldwork opportunities.

To be a useful approach for day-release training, PBL does not have to be an all-or-none choice. With adjustments it may be incorporated into the weekly programme alongside existing features. What needs to be established is whether it is possible to provide a sufficiently broad range of learning within the confines of the course, given that each topic requires two lengthy group sessions as well as befores and afters. The prospect of real expansion of usable day-release time through longer training practice attachments should make possible the implementation of PBL as a core method in vocational training.

Pulling it together

How do the overall aims and objectives of the course fit together to constitute a programme for the term, the year and the whole three-year course? The variety of the component parts is potentially endless. They range, in structure, from short episodes of self-resourced group discussion to major modules extending over weeks; in setting, from classroom to fieldwork; and in method, from individual assignments to symposia.

The weekly programme requires a flexible framework on which to hang things (*see* Figures 2.1 and 2.2). Allowance must be made for special events which do not readily fit the normal template: a session of fieldwork, e.g. visiting a factory or prison, requires planning which is dictated by the nature of the event. Day-release time is short and each item on the programme is a specific learning exercise rather than a slot to be filled.

Preparing the term's programme comes as an early challenge to the new course organizer. It is important not to get bogged down in it but to see it as an administrative exercise with educational overtones. It is sensible to leave gaps for unfinished business and to allow trainees to get involved in shaping curriculum content. Keep an eye on the overall year plan – it is frustrating to reach the final term and find that not everything can be crammed in.

Have a statement of *aims* for every component and some indication of how you will assess the extent to which they were met. This may involve simple report sheets similar to those shown in Figures 6.1 and 6.2.

The *content* of your programme will be guided by suggestions from the trainees and trainers, and awareness of the major themes, tasks and methods of primary care and other current issues.

The *methods* should reflect your interpretation of learner-centredness and process orientation. This may mean opting for group-interactive and action-learning approaches, or employing the widest possible range of methods in each component for the sake of variety while sensing what works for your particular group. With time you will become more selective about the methods you choose for a given situation.

The *resources* you need to employ should be at the service of the aims, content and methods. The chief resources are yourself and the trainees. By the time each session starts, the bulk of your educational contribution may already have been made. Do as little as possible of the didactic work yourself. Involve the trainees in resourcing sessions at every level: preparing and sharing information, and hosting and chairing sessions. Involve GPs (especially the trainers) as resource persons at every opportunity, but also invite non-medical resource people where possible – they often see things differently and bring a fresh perspective. Consultants and other medical specialists may have an important contribution to make, especially if they are carefully chosen and clearly briefed. Question-and-answer sessions are useful to ensure that specialist expertise is matched with learners' needs. Another approach is to use the invited resource person as a commentator on the material prepared and presented by trainees themselves. If the group invite an external resource person, they are entitled to say what is needed.

Preparing the programme is then a matter of timetabling. One method is to start with a large sheet of A1 paper (flip chart size). Divide it in two along the axis, and then divide the lower half into columns corresponding to the number of days in the term. Block off those days which are outside your discretion, e.g. assessment points, scheme meetings and residentials. Treat the upper half similarly. In each upper column, list the activities, events and topics you wish to include. Match upper and lower columns according to themes, availability of invited resource people, priorities, educational content and methods, aiming to achieve in each session a balance between structured and unstructured work.

The following list may help you to prepare and assess elements of the course.

Guidelines

Where possible, the curriculum should:

- be learner sensitive
- sample the curriculum rather than cover it
- focus on root and stem rather than branch, twig and leaf
- empower rather than inform, demonstrating principles and methods which may be generalized
- explore knowledge, concepts and values; encourage an evidence-based approach; have 'process' as well as 'content' aims
- have a statement of aims and corresponding assessment methods
- be based on more than one educational method, using variety to promote involvement
- be as participatory as possible involving preparation and presentation by (some) trainees
- involve resource persons who are well briefed about their role and the methods to be used within the session.

The evaluation cycle

Successful curriculum development incorporates self-righting mechanisms. Unless there is systematic evaluation built into the course and its individual elements, there may be a curriculum but no development. The evaluation of curriculum items is among your chief learning tools as a course organizer. Each time you conduct a teaching exercise it is an experiment – a test of the educational hypothesis enshrined in your aims. Take the opportunity to write down observations and conclusions and, having done so, do not just file and forget them.

The following questions may be useful, even if subjective:

- what did the learners think of it?
- what did I think of it?
- what did the resource person think of it?
- was it worth it?
- what should be done differently next time?
- how valid are the responses to these questions?

Of all the questions, the last is the most significant. Most course organizers know of excellent contributions which are given the thumbs down for the wrong reason. All trainees know of the negative feelings they suppress in order to avoid conflict or hurting the course organizer's feelings. Evaluation can be made more valid by specific questioning such as:

- can you identify two things you learned from today's presentation?
- in what way do you now feel differently towards… ?
- in what way will today's presentation influence your actions when you are consulting?

In some situations more complex evaluation procedures are productive, for example:

- reflection on outcomes after a period of time indicates whether new knowledge resulted in a changed state
- groupwork exercises as a follow-up produce evidence through observation of content, process and task completion
- questionnaires and short-answer papers on topics covered.

Much of Chapter 6 is relevant to the evaluation cycle of curriculum development.

Who is teaching whom?

Learner-centredness is not just for the benefit of the trainees: it is also a protection for the course organizer. If you begin by regarding yourself as the teacher, you place yourself at risk of certain hazards:

- the trap of omniscience
- the trap of omnicompetence
- the 'Guru syndrome', inviting dependence by inhibiting the trainees' development as autonomous learners
- the 'God syndrome', trying to create beings 'in your own image and likeness' (*Genesis*, 1.27).

You are confronted with the limitations of your own abilities. Identifying with the learners blurs the teacher–learner axis, and enables your learning and that of the trainees to grow at the same time. Therefore the learning curriculum for you as a course organizer should in turn influence the process by which the group will learn. Freire (1972) was the most eminent exponent of the action-reflection model of learning which has more recently been reinterpreted by Schön (1983) in his advocacy of reflection-in-action. In curriculum terms this means reflecting on questions such as:

- what do I wish to learn as a practising GP?
- what skills do I need to meet my own learning needs?
- what situations do I meet in practice that baffle me or make my heart sink?

These provide the basis for your learning curriculum as a professional and indicate the sort of authentic and effective learning situations you should provide for the trainees. The chief danger in this approach – the 'God syndrome' – is averted by the extent to which you respect the learners, evaluate your efforts and submit them to the discernment of your peers.

The most challenging concept in developing a curriculum is that of ensuring that doctors are capable of managing their own learning for the remaining 30 years or so of their professional lives. The emphasis of the course organizer must therefore be on modelling for the trainees the ability to be continually self-learning.

'Vocational training cannot provide all the skills and knowledge necessary for the remainder of a professional career.' (RCGP, 1990)

Exercise 13

As a continuing learner yourself you should be able to prepare a programme for communicating to the trainees the knowledge, concepts, values and methodology of continuing learning. Why not try it?

Summary

It is not difficult to find sound theoretical guidance concerning the curriculum of vocational training, beginning with the Leeuwenhorst formulation of the job description of the generic European family physician. The problem for the course organizer is how to identify the learning priorities in practice, and what methods and resources to employ to supplement those of the training practice and hospital settings.

The aim of this chapter has been to delineate the principles that will enable the course organizer to choose appropriately from the extensive published lists of educational contents and methods. It is suggested that the focus should be on:

- mapping the territory of general practice knowledge
- sampling relevant aspects of general practice
- avoiding those elements which can be done better in other settings
- involving trainees in achieving an overview of their own professional development
- focusing on topics which ramify in content and method, and generalizing from these to achieve transferable skills and knowledge
- co-ordinating learning situations which enable trainees to integrate their increasing knowledge with appropriate concepts and values
- assessing progress in ways which identify further learning needs and indicate ways of improving the learning experience.

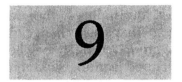

9

The perspective of the learning continuum

Introduction: Pilgrim's progress

The education chapters have focused on the course organizer, the group of trainees and the process of vocational training. This is a limited, if necessary, perspective – especially on the initial slopes of the course organizer's learning curve. However, it is a useful maxim in training not to lose sight of the finished product.

What is the 'finished product' of GP vocational training? The chapters on assessment dealt with landmarks and goals through the vocational training scheme. Earlier chapters outlined concepts and equipment that might be needed for planning and starting out on the 'journey' with the trainee group. Chapters subsequent to this one address the cohesion of the pilgrims on the way and some logistic support for the expedition leader.

At this point, approximately half way through the book, it is necessary to call a halt, to see how far you have come, to take sightings for the way ahead and to practise using some gear that might be needed in the steeper, more isolated, changing territory that lies ahead.

The finished product is a mature, autonomous, continuing learner.

The learning continuum

'Give a man a fish, you feed him for today; he will be happy. Teach him to fish, he may argue with you now but he will survive.' (Adapted proverb)

No section on education would be complete unless placed in the context of lifelong learning. Much emphasis has been placed on the trainees as adult learners – however, many trainees do not seem to fit the adult learner mould. Older trainees who are undertaking vocational training at a more than average age, perhaps as a change in career path, find difficulty in acclimatizing to the day-release group setting. It may be a matter of age gap or role transition, but there is also a structured learning situation which makes demands reminiscent of undergraduate days (or even school). The classroom situation, the examinations, assignments, formative assessment exercises all contradict the image of the autonomous learner who embraces further learning for its own sake. Anyone re-entering training having been an autonomous professional experiences as much difficulty as those who 'enter from below'. A balance between pedagogy and androgogy must be recognized and handled with sensitivity.

Trainees are in a transitional learning phase. In developmental terms it is an adolescence in professional life which may explain occasional turbulent behaviour. This suggests the developmental perceptive of tolerating regression while laying the groundwork for lifelong autonomy.

What does this mean in practical course-organizing terms? There are tasks to be completed, examinations to be passed. The approach of pedagogy has much to contribute to this and the structured learning exercise, lecture and coursework can provide a reassuringly familiar feel. The approach of androgogy (adult learning) makes more demands on teacher and learner. A gradual transition from one to the other would be helpful, but the timing of examinations hinders this. So there has to be a dual approach.

I think it is important that the trainees' co-operation in this transition is enlisted. Along with clinical and management skills they should become skilled in their approach to continuing education – the management of their future continuing professional development (CPD). This raises a dilemma. Educational theory is tedious enough for those who need to know it. Clinicians seem to be particularly irritated by it and it is difficult material to teach. However, can they become adequate managers of their CPD without knowing anything about it? Thousands will happily answer 'Yes'! The alternative, less populist, view is that doctors are managers of information. They acquire it and impart it. They can do either well and consciously or take their chances in ignorance. I prefer the alternative view and propose that trainee GPs should learn about learning and teaching.

'The fundamental process of learning to learn is that of taking over and internalising the functions of the teacher/trainer; of learning to do for oneself what others have, hitherto, done for one.' (Squires, 1994)

Learning how to learn

The assertion that human beings are inherently self-educating given the right circumstances (Neighbour, 1987) has the ring of truth about it. However, running is inherent but many people do not bother to do it, let alone try to run better.

Most third-level students on arrival at university find that the induction process offers workshops on study skills. Uptake of this is low; they must think they already know how. However, as they progress towards finals they become increasingly aware that their learning is impeded by their difficulty in assimilating and applying the quantity of knowledge they are faced with.

The final year of vocational training is a learning challenge on all fronts – knowledge, skills, capabilities and competence. The assessments are wide-ranging and searching. If it is possible to enhance the capacity to learn quickly and effectively this would be a worthy starting point.

An initial problem is resistance from the learners. They are impatient to get to grips with clinical practice material and they resent this apparent deviation into unfamiliar territory and may feel they have nothing to gain from it, having got this far without it. However, a few simple exercises may help change their mind. Exercises 14 and 15 aim to explore cognitive dissonance, a powerful tool for opening up areas of knowledge where learner resistance is anticipated. It operates through uncovering gaps, misperceptions and learning needs.

Exercise 14 deals with how trainees use medical journals by asking them to indicate their priorities on the contents page of a current journal edition. Responses frequently indicate a wide range in the number of journal articles selected and variety of topics addressed. Some will be sparing in their choice, some will mark a huge number of items for detailed reading. The discussion often reveals that they select according to key words on a basis of empathy with the topic and a predisposition towards clinical content in keeping with the years of experience in a hospital setting. This should be challenged with reference to the community setting – what does it say to the GP?

Many trainees use journals like coffee-table magazines – to browse superficially and leave. Many do not receive their own copy of a journal regularly. This limits their options for storing and retrieving material and few are likely to be practising a systematic method for doing this. The outcome may produce guidelines such as:

- subscribe to the *British Medical Journal* and the *British Journal of General Practice*
- start a filing system arranged in subject files and collect clippings/photocopies
- start a subject index on filing cards with summaries of useful data, indexed to source
- scan journals for key words relevant to general practice content and method.

The underlying strategy is to discover that they do not know what they don't know and that the beginning of learning is a needs assessment, a map of the areas they need to explore and methods to consolidate learning. Existing notions of what constitutes adequate, useful knowledge may have to be discarded or adapted to a new setting.

Exercise 14

How do you use medical journals? Targeting items.

Materials   Flipchart; copy and distribute the contents page of a recent *BMJ*.

Instructions Underline the items you would read in detail. Put a cross at those where you would read the summary only.

Process   Tabulate on flipchart and discuss differences in selection.

• How do you read journals: when and where? Group discussion: each group member says how he uses medical journals, how often and in what setting? Discuss the variety of answers.
• Outcomes: how much do you retain from reading a medical journal? Group discussion: ask each group member to think of an item read recently and outline its content. Discuss any problems experienced in this process.
• How do you recall, store or retrieve information derived from reading journals? Write down a shortlist of methods. Group discussion: using flipchart, list the answers, brainstorm on other ways.
• Summarize guidelines for storing/retrieving information.

Exercise 15

Group discussion: What is your treatment of a child with a sore ear?

• Now go to the library and carry out a literature search on the words 'otitis media – treatment'. Note down number of references, but do not print out.
• What problems do you encounter in carrying out this task?

Exercise 15 is a group discussion of a common clinical problem – the child with a sore ear which at first sight is simple. Discussion may ramify from 'painkillers and an antibiotic' to encompass concepts like differential diagnosis of ear pain, the natural history of otitis media, the bacteriological evidence that guides therapy, the concept of the catarrhal child, the effectiveness of antibiotics versus other approaches, practice policies on antibiotic use. If they do not get there, a few cues will reveal the problems. Then, do they know how to find out answers to the questions that arise without drowning in printout and costing the library a fortune?

This should not be seen as an attempt to humiliate the learner, but to motivate towards change and bring it about. This is helped by the clear message that the goals of change can be identified, the tasks involved defined, the skills explained and demonstrated, and the appropriate resources made available.

The next step is to show that learning is not a linear process. It happens at various levels – cognitive, affective and behavioural; through a variety of means – active and passive, individual and group based; in a variety of settings – in the practice, at home, in the library, with the group; and it is subject to an assessment cycle which opens up new questions. Learning has to be purposeful and consolidated by recording or putting it into practice in altered behaviour. Thus, it is an active process combining knowledge, action and reflection, goal setting and assessment.

An extension of this is the construction of *learning templates* which provide a structured approach to thinking through different situations:

- any chronic disease can be managed by creating a generalizable approach derived from discussing a few chronic diseases such as diabetes, asthma or rheumatoid arthritis
- a small number of different templates can be constructed which will cover most MEQ-type questions
- any critical appraisal task can be approached by using an appropriate set of headings
- the evidence base for a clinical question can be constructed by the use of structured thinking such as:
  - how do I manage x in the surgery and why?
  - how did I arrive at this approach?
  - is there public policy on this?
  - are there official report data published?
  - are there guidelines published by a reputable interest group?

These exercises should result in effective learning about the chosen topic and this should help convince them that 'learning to learn' is worthwhile.

More about learning how to learn

Having, hopefully, addressed resistance to the concept of educational theory it is important not to get carried away by 'educationalism'. What do they need to know and how to convey it in a productive way? They need just enough for them to organize themselves properly. This can be achieved through a number of exercises which are rooted in clinical learning but where the underlying learning theory can be made explicit through reflecting on and discussing the attendant processes. These can be summed up as:

- needs assessment
- learning styles

- goal setting
- information technology
- problem-based learning
- drawing conclusions for continuing learning.

Try to avoid lecturing about educational theory and instead demonstrate it in the course of interesting clinical or problem-solving exercises.

Needs assessment

Needs assessment should not be unfamiliar to trainees but should be emphasized as a fundamental element of all postgraduate education. Early use of checklists, multiple choice and modified essay question papers, analysis of random cases or video-recorded consultations will reveal much of the curriculum to be addressed and invite their curiosity to identify areas of new learning.

Learning styles

Learning styles may be an unfamiliar concept which merits a specific exploratory approach. Its importance lies in exploring the individuals' differing approaches to carrying out tasks, helping them to value their preferred approach while perceiving a challenge to expand their repertoire of study skills and ability to gain from different learning environments. This can be approached through the use of various psycho-metric tools (well-known ones include Myers – Briggs (1962), Riding (1994), Honey and Mumford (1992)). It may be useful to employ a local educational psychologist to resource a seminar/workshop. This helps towards some practical ends such as:

- showing why some are natural 'groupies' while others have difficulty with learning in groups, thereby resolving the feeling of good or bad group members
- insight into use of time – the complementary nature of 'hard' and 'soft' knowledge and tolerance of the different timeframe appropriate to assimilating factual stuff from that needed to address skills or feelings
- appreciation of teamwork issues – the value of differing personalities' contribution to a group practice or committee (the *ideas generator* may not be the best person to *carry out* a decision)
- grasp of communication problems with patients – why different doctors find different patients difficult; why a health education task may have to be modified to take account of patients' different cognitive styles
- help with selecting the most effective approach to learning for each member in the group. This may affect the course organizer's selection of teaching–learning methods.

One way of realizing this is to run a workshop based around health education. As a preparatory task each member should prepare a simple health education exercise enlisting the help of their training practice team members. It should define the message to be imparted, identify the target group, the medium and materials to be used and speculate about how its effectiveness would be assessed. A member of the local Health Promotion Unit might be asked to resource the presentations at the day-release course analysing the cognitive/educational issues which arise. The difference between, for example, verbalizers and visualizers (script-writers *v* diagram-drawers) should become evident (*see* Chapter 11).

Goal setting

It is a dogma of vocational training that the trainees should be involved in decisions about the content of the day-release course. They need facilitation in this for three reasons.

1 They may never have been involved before in determining the course of their own learning.
2 There is a tendency to give superficial answers 'off the top of the head' when invited to set goals.
3 Weakness in goal setting is reflected in trite comments which characterize most feedback sheets returned at the end of day-release course (and CME) sessions.

If learners are only dimly aware of what they ought to be learning who can fault them for vaguely and superficially assessing the effectiveness of what they gain from learning situations? Effort invested in goal setting contributes to formative assessment, evaluation and appraisal.

Asking trainees what they want to achieve and to outline the tasks that bring this about is a starting point which ought to be revisited periodically. Greater depth is achievable through group activities aimed at allowing individuals to clarify for themselves their aims and values, gaps and weak points.

* reflecting on the strengths and weaknesses of their educational experiences to date to identify what helped or hindered
* talking about their reasons for wanting to be GPs
* describing 'icon figures' and how they were influenced by them ('the person who most influenced my career path...')
* life-mapping exercises to identify directions, goals and turning points in life experience and what was learned from these, e.g. 'I did not enjoy medical school. As a SHO everything seemed to go downhill. The turning point was a post in psychiatry. The next high point was my first few weeks as a registrar in the training practice. Then our first baby arrived and I had to review my priorities'

- creation of vision statements or symbolic representations related to career and vocation, e.g. a poster, heraldic shield, poem
- drawing up a wish list of items for the programme, e.g. 'I would like to visit a hospice, learn how to use e-mail'
- giving feedback to one another concerning perceived abilities and strengths. This stimulates both the group and the respective recipient member to privately identify their own strengths and weaknesses: 'I wish I had Jo's ability to defuse tension in the group and her presentation skills'.

Tabulating outcomes of these exercises should lead to a priority list. It will not be possible to realize them all during the day-release course but individuals can carry away ideas for follow-up with their trainer or by private exploration. This should also contribute to periodic individual appraisal with the course organizer which is another useful approach to goal setting.

Clearly, not all of this can or should be completed in the first week of the day-release course. It should begin early but it is yet another cyclical process characteristic of education.

Information technology

This used to be called the library. It would be as wrong to assume that all young doctors know a lot about computers as to assume that older doctors know how to use a medical library. Most people use their available technology superficially, e.g. one programme on the washing machine, and few get the opportunity to overcome their instinctive blocks and make breakthroughs into sophisticated use of what is available. A workshop run by a medical librarian is a useful start. It should include the use of manual indexes, databases, resource shelves in the library and the location of relevant sections in the stack. Then the automated bits make more sense. Encounters with the modern tools should include individual hands-on tasks using microfiche, CD-ROM, on-line search and the Internet.

This opens up to the individual the possibility of autonomous learning which is the basis of continuing medical education (CME). Hopefully they will not forget the basics, like occasionally getting out a book and reading it.

Problem-based learning

Problem-based learning (*see also* Chapters 5 and 8) enables the learners to combine group and individual skills, clinical and methodology training, critical thinking, presentation skills and familiarity with the literature on topics addressed. It has been shown to have lasting influence on learning behaviour, and you cannot say much better than that for any educational approach.

- 'My preferred learning style is...'
- 'I learn most effectively by...'
- 'My weakest learning style is...'
- 'I will work on it by...'
- 'My approach to needs assessment is...'
- 'What attracts me least about the curriculum is...'
- 'I will approach this by...'
- 'The tasks I need to focus on are...'
- 'My approach to "journal club activities" ought to be...'
- 'My system for recording and retrieving data is based on...'
- 'My study timetable is...'
- 'One thing I want to achieve by the end of the year...'

Figure 9.1 Outline of personal learning contract.

Drawing conclusions

Drawing conclusions is a necessary outcome of action/reflection. If the 'learning how to learn module' so far described has any impact, it is through trying out the various bits, derived as they may be from theoretical constructs, and discovering what works. Unfortunately this cannot be prescribed, it ought to be specific to each individual in the group despite much common ground and should address the whole area of CME. As an experiment it is worthwhile asking the trainees to attend a small number of CME activities, preferably self-selected, local and ordinary. A group discussion can then analyse the features of the events and devise profiles of what makes for a good or bad CME event and speculate about the effect of other kinds of settings or approaches.

Conclusions may then be drawn up by each trainee in the form of a personal educational contract or manifesto as shown in Figure 9.1.

Using what you know

All practitioners, especially those in training, should develop a respect for their existing knowledge base. This is particularly important in practical problem solving and in doing examinations. It is the best starting point for combating a feeling of helplessness or hopelessness in the face of a daunting situation – be it a consultation or examination question. General practice exists within limitless boundaries and a knowledge requirement that can never be comprehensive. At all career stages we bring to bear on whatever situation we meet a repertoire of knowledge including basic sciences, clinical medicine, life experience and back-up resources that can be accessed. Therefore an insoluble problem should be rare. When faced with an unfamiliar problem or a lack of specific knowledge use your 'know how' to supplement your 'know what'.

Guidelines for using what you know in an examination

- Start with what you already know and write it down.
- Brainstorm to create a flow of ideas.
- Think yourself into the situation ('mental role-play').
- Generate alternative approaches, e.g. management plans and templates.
- Identify the blocks to progress.
- Note how you would attack these through using databases, teamwork or other resources, such as by referral.
- Scan your memory for help: the discriminating use of
  - particularizing from the general
  - generalizing from the particular
  - applying first principles.

The trainee should never have to turn in a blank page in response to any examination question.

Unlearning and dumping

Anyone who uses a database, be it manual or electronic, soon encounters the problem of clutter. Retrieving information is hindered by the very accumulation of items. The physical solution is regular weeding and shredding or deletion. Files may have to be reorganized under different headings where there is a significant problem about where new material belongs.

So it is with learning. Information overload is a familiar concept and one historical response is to rely on the existing stock of information and ignore the flood of contributing, often conflicting, information. This has obvious dangers. Strategies for unlearning include:

- developing the perspective of continuing learning; emphasize the range of CME activities
- developing the skills of evidence-based practice
- regular practice of audit

- review of personal sources of data, discarding old textbooks, old journal clippings, old items from a subject-indexed file system
- regularly updating these data sources: new documents in your 'store' should be dated and source-referenced for later review, updating or dumping
- occasional needs assessment in areas that do not really interest you but might be important
- tuning in to cognitive dissonance.

All this is quite compatible with having a historical perspective on the development of ideas in a given field. Unlearning does not excuse amnesia. It involves change in practice and belief systems in the light of authenticated perspective (Wilson, 1988). Examples:

- GP registrars, following their transition from hospital to the community, will need to review familiar management plans for certain conditions like 'chest pain' or 'headache' in view of the difference in setting, prevalence, technological back-up and the different power relationship between doctor and patient in primary care. Some personality types will have difficulty with this and may need help with developing lateral thinking to supplement linear approaches.
- The Prochaska–di Clemente (1986) cycle of behaviour change in addiction throws new light on the management of smoking cessation, alcoholism and related behaviours. Do people still have to reach 'rock bottom' before they can be helped to change? Can we therefore continue to adopt a position of hopelessness in relation to addicts? What is the evidence for regarding alcoholism as a 'disease'?

Dumping old evidence in favour of the new marks a change in knowledge. To change further, in attitudes and behaviour, involves openness to change, challenging rigidity, tuning in to cognitive dissonance, abandoning obsolete practices and replacing the misleading with the enlightened. This may be liberating in opening up new perspectives and allowing time-consuming and inappropriate tasks to be identified and dumped but unfortunately there are not enough of these to compensate for the new tasks accumulating in primary care. Learning skills in delegation and management will help. Example:

- Running cervical cytology, asthma and diabetic clinics diverts much time from the open availability of doctors' time. Skill in team development, the use of evidence-based protocols, audit and appraisal may release doctor-time by allowing a nurse and a secretary to operate this system with in-built clinical safeguards.

Learning problem solving and decision making

Problem solving is a basic activity of all practitioners. In Schön's (1983) view, practitioners 'manage messes'. They try to bring order into the soft boggy territory of human situations, at two removes from the high, firm ground of the pure scientist (applied scientists occupying the territory between). Where the scientists function by eliminating variables, practitioners accept that real situations have multiple variables and intervene by trying to reduce complex reality to a number of manageable problems. This involves observation, reflection and problem setting. Brainstorming contributes to this process by generating ideas which can then be prioritized and hypotheses that can be tested. Where a major decision has to be made a technique called SWOT analysis can be applied. This acronym stands for:

Strengths
Weaknesses
Opportunities
Threats.

Normally used in corporate planning it is applicable to policy decisions in practice management and to some crucial clinical decision making.

Other aids to problem solving lie in the area of audit. Conventional clinical audit is an essential part of the training curriculum and is considered elsewhere (*see* Part 5). A more recent extension of this is critical incident analysis or significant event auditing and a detailed report has been published by the RCGP (Pringle *et al.,* 1995). In essence a significant event, e.g. a patient dying or a complaint, is subjected to peer scrutiny in a supportive way which allows in-depth analysis of the circumstances and perceptions of the key workers, identifies learning points and recommends changes in the clinical or management approach to address the risk of recurrence. This kind of activity, related to the work of hospital mortality committees, can be a potent educational and administrative tool (McEvoy, 1975).

Related concepts include *risk analysis* which identifies the probability of adverse consequences arising from a given situation or course of action, and *decision theory* which deals with the use of decision trees in choosing between options (Gau, 1994).

A final safety net in the problem-solving/decision-making complex is *help-seeking strategies*. Every interviewing panel wishes to examine the candidate's insight into the boundaries of role and competence, and the ability to know when and how to seek help. Examples of help seeking include consulting colleagues, practice meeting, team meeting, use of allied professions, referral to specialist, consulting sources of further information, specific interest groups (many of them disease specific, such as the British Diabetic Association) and consulting professional bodies, e.g. defence organization, regional advisers, etc.

Pulling it together

This chapter began by posing the question – what is the finished product of vocational training? This can be answered at two levels:

1 a qualified competent candidate for a GP principal post
2 as above, with additional qualities like empathy and self-insight and equipped to manage his or her own professional development.

The first level is the common ground. This is addressed by core curriculum topics and summative assessment. The second level involves 'higher order' teaching and learning skills. None of us comes with an inbuilt blueprint for this whether we are the teachers or the learners. The early chapters of Part 2 addressed level one attainments for trainee and course organizer. This chapter has attempted to open up level two and there is a dynamic and growing body of literature to further assist this (*see* Part 6).

Elegance in consulting, therapeutics and management are attainments on a life-long scale. The neglected interface between vocational training and professional life lies in the area of skills for continuing professional development and awareness of the discipline of education is central to addressing this interface.

Education is a strange subject and resembles computer science. Who wants to know what goes on in the mother board, disk drive and programmes when what they need to do is type a document? However, those who use the capacity of their PC to best effect, including when things go wrong or a new kind of task is required, are those who know something about the workings of the technology. This technology draws on many fields of knowledge.

Educational technology is not a pure science, but an applied one at the service of the practitioners. It remains a largely derivative discipline (Squires, 1994) and it would be unrealistic to expect GP teachers or learners to be deeply versed in it. What is needed is a working knowledge. A good theorist is not the same as a good practitioner – however, Squires maintains that if you 'scratch a practitioner you will find a theorist'. A competent practitioner (teacher) will wish to convey to the client (learner) enough insight to serve the client's needs – but only enough. It is counter-productive to draw the client into the web of concepts, decisions and value-judgements that underlie the praxis. What is needed is educational common sense.

'The greater the difficulty the lecturer has in keeping the audience awake, the more likely is the lecture to be about educational technique.' (O'Donnell, 1986)

This is the daunting task of the medical educator – to balance health care priorities with educational idealism in fostering the trainee practitioner's growth towards professional maturity. There is no direct evidence to show what works in the long term. In the absence of the possibility of demonstrated validity we must proceed with training for continuing professional development on the basis of face validity.

To facilitate education towards CPD it is important for the course organizer to be familiar with the issues and growth points in continuing medical education. There is a great and growing literature and the following distillation of CME is drawn from a recent overview of CME in the UK (McEvoy, 1997).

CME in a nutshell

- CME is an obligation of professionalism – a core value.
- It should be determined by the practitioner on the basis of needs assessment.
- It is not about re-certification but is a voluntary growth exercise.
- Learning that does not challenge does not effect change.
- Active learning is better than passive learning.
- Most CME events rely on passive learning – there is little evidence of its value.
- Other values co-exist in CME – socialization, morale and networking.
- It should have an interdisciplinary perspective.
- It requires protected time, realistic pricing and positive incentives.
- It requires reflection, evaluation and follow-up.
- Portfolio-based learning, Balint (and other) groups, mentoring, audit, research and taking higher degrees are increasingly recognized as productive approaches.
- CPD may stand for both continuing development of the practitioner and continuing development of the profession.
- Learning should rely on purposeful and continuing processes rather than on discrete and arbitrary events.
- It should embody the following values:
  - stimulation of scientific and intellectual curiosity
  - revitalization and channelling of creative energy
  - enhancement of professionalism
  - empowerment towards innovation and change
  - avoidance of professional and personal stagnation, isolation and burnout.

Part 3

The course organizer
and group work

Overview

The aim of the two chapters which make up Part 3 is to provide a rationale for group work in the day-release course. A course organizer may regard himself as a trainer who has a group instead of a trainee, and he must therefore explore and develop the potential of the group just as the trainer would the registrar. The basic terminology is explained and the characteristics of the group setting are described. This sets the scene for Chapter 11, which introduces some of the functions, rules and exercises appropriate to the course organizer as he begins to explore the educational potential of the day-release course group.

Like education and management, the theory of groups has to be tested and tried in real life to have any value, and it is usually the theoretical aspect that has to be flexible to meet the practicalities. The scenario shows that theory is a way of making sense of reality and this creates feelings for the leader, and it is with the feelings of course organizers that Chapter 10 begins.

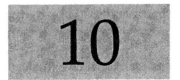

10

Group work

Introduction

'The most stressful thing for me about working in groups is the constant uncertainty about how it will go and whether it will fail for some participants and that I may not recognize it.' (Anonymous course organizer)

The survey of the needs and problems identified by course organizers in their early days (*see* Chapter 1) revealed some insecurity about leading group work. The anxieties centred on the lack of experience in groups, uncertainty about the place of group work in the vocational training scheme and fear of damaging people in the group setting. For most new course organizers it is clearly a threatening and unfamiliar activity.

Doctors react very differently to the idea of group work. It is likely to appeal more to extroverts than to introverts, to 'feelers' rather than to 'thinkers'. Reactions do not determine ability or effectiveness, but negative reactions do have to be recognized and dealt with. This applies equally to course organizer and trainee.

Most of us have attitudes somewhere between those of the keen groupie and the rationalist sceptic; and most people approach the prospect of leading a group with apprehension. The following comments are typical:

- *'I'm afraid of making a fool of myself in front of a bunch of sceptical trainees'*
- *'I'm afraid of drying up or "freezing" in the middle of some unstructured group exercise'*
- *'I'm afraid of failure'*
- *'My GP colleagues might think me foolish'*
- *'My kite might not get off the ground when everyone else's kite is soaring'*
- *'I'm afraid of the unknown'*

The vast majority of course organizers admit to having had such fears, and not all the anxieties ever go away completely. However, most course organizers who attend courses in group training find it enjoyable, stimulating and liberating. They get to know themselves better and handle crises better as a result. They find that they can speed up their trainees' learning by helping them to lower their barriers. They regret the loss of opportunity when a group of trainees sits passively through a lesson which they could have got in a library any time.

Group work can be deeply satisfying and course organizers want to share this opportunity with generations of trainees, knowing that they will, in turn, carry out more elegant consultations, handle meetings with staff and colleagues more effectively and get more job satisfaction from their professional life.

However, group work has to be introduced and implemented with sensitivity. It helps if you start by facing up to your own feelings about it. People often have surprisingly strong subconscious feelings on the subject. The more you know about and experience the realities of group work, the less of an obstacle these will be. Attending an introductory course on group work is a good start.

Demystifying group work

Few educational activities are more shrouded in mystique. Demystifying it is a useful starting place. As a course organizer you will not be conducting group psychotherapy or an unstructured 'California-style feel-in'. Nor will you be leading a group of passive subjects deep into their collective unconscious. Leading group work is not a performance you put on for the trainees. You are more likely to have to stop a heated discussion because the trainee group has overrun its time on the journal club, or have to help the quietest member express opinions, or summarize the gist of a debate about the ethics of screening. Not everything that happens in a group is group work, but there are group work elements to everything that happens when people get together. The course organizer's role is to discern and address the group's needs and to encourage discovery in a protected atmosphere of trust.

Definitions

A *group* is a small number of people who embark on a common task together. A *task* is a formulation of the overt objectives of the group, while *process* refers to everything that goes on in the group as it pursues its overt task.

Group work, whilst literally meaning very little, is here understood to mean the deliberate and skilful co-ordination of a small number of consenting people in a learning activity in which both task and process are expected to have educative value.

Process group work takes place when the analysis of process issues is defined as the immediate task.

While leadership roles and activities may be performed by various group participants from time to time and leadership is a function of the group as a whole, the task of group leadership is usually vested in an identified member of the group. *Maintenance, management, boundary holding* and *climate building* are ways in which the leader fosters the group's ability to carry out tasks effectively.

Feedback refers to the verbal and non-verbal messages each member receives about himself from the group or any member in the group setting.

There is a multitude of terms to describe roles and behaviours in group work, many of which are illustrated in an entertaining book of cartoons and descriptions by Kindred (1995).

Why group work? Its place in vocational training

The course organizer is a trainer to a group of trainees. It would be as much a dereliction for the course organizer to neglect the identity and well-being of the group as for the trainer to ignore the individuality of the trainee. If the potential of the group situation is not recognized and managed, we might as well have distance learning courses. (These are not inferior, just different.) It is frequently asserted that our behaviour in groups reflects our behaviour at work or in consultation. The group setting facilitates learning activities which are less accessible in other contexts, e.g. pooling of information, co-operative task work, discussion of problems, ventilation of feeling, mutual support, modelling, self-assessment, broadening of perspectives and exploration of why people perceive, react and behave differently. It is a bridge between *cognitive* and *experiential* learning, between how we think and how we feel or behave.

Who are the group?

When people get together in small group work, they constitute a new 'organism' with its own natural history. It may be regarded in terms of its anatomy, physiology, pathology and 'higher functions'. Its organs are represented by the individuals. Its identity is defined by boundaries related to size, purpose and desire to belong. It also demonstrates phenomena akin to immunity – rejection of foreign bodies or influences which are not compatible with it – and occasionally auto-immunity!

A gathering such as the day-release course may not constitute a single organic entity. Complexities arise because of members entering at different times, erratic attendance and differing levels of consent, stages of professional development and numbers involved. The purposes or agendas will vary from time to time, resulting in regrouping or subdividing. It is not a simple organism, but a dynamic interaction of people, task and process. It follows that subgroups may need to be discerned and differentiated, coalesced or wound up. This organism's life cycle is further considered in Chapter 11.

What group work?

Why do course organizers not just organize speakers for the day-release course programme, as their name implies?

We all do some of that since every course has set pieces which need to be covered. That model was a necessary and fruitful phase in the evolution of course organizing. Experience has shown that deliberately moving the proceedings to and fro, along the line between task and process orientation, changes the depth and quality of learning.

The group work approach is not necessarily about doing different things but about doing things differently. It entails inviting people into their own learning process, using their own experiences and relating to one another actively. A traditional teaching setting can allow these features to develop. The major difference between the two settings relates to the use of power. Who makes the decisions and how are they reached?

Many productive small group activities are based on fairly conventional tasks like case discussion (random case analysis, Balint group), exploring a theme (e.g. ethics, management, prevention) and developing and practising skills (learning consultation skills using videos of one's own consultations, problem-based learning).

How the group sees these activities depends on how much has been invested in developing the levels of communication, trust and co-operation that the group members bring to these tasks and the nature of the agreements that underlie their approach.

More personally challenging, perhaps, are the kinds of group exercises where members share experiences from their own non-professional lives, practise communication skills, role-play problems to explore varieties of outcome, brainstorm on dilemmas or explore decision making through negotiation (*see* Chapter 11).

These activities require planning and sometimes rehearsal by the leader away from the group setting. Particular materials may also be needed. The group work approach is not an excuse for having no programme, plans or props. Tasks are important. If the group lacks a clear agreed task, process takes over. This is not a bad thing, if you are prepared for it and know how to help people learn through examination of process issues.

There are group settings where learning through the process is at least as valuable as achieving the overt task. Where there is convergence of the two, where the exploration and appreciation of the *process* is the *task*, we have *process group work*. This is particularly useful in developing interpersonal skills, sensitivity towards others, insight into one's own behaviour and awareness of what is going on amongst interacting individuals. This can be time consuming and emotionally charged, and it demands skilled leadership.

There is a perceptible gradient of skills required as you move from task to process. Avoid extremes, either playing it so safe that nothing moves out of the 'task station', or heading down the line so fast that you'll crash into the buffers at the 'process station'.

Assessing the extent to which the group tasks were achieved is an important aspect of any conscious group exercise: whether learning took place, process issues were identified and resolved, what the experience meant to participants and whether there is any unfinished business. The leader should watch for signs of distress in any individual, as these may indicate personal unfinished business. This may need to be dealt with after the session is over. In the words of Hopson and Scally (1981): *'The more Befores and Afters you have the better your teaching is likely to be.'*

Group work: when?

Group work begins when a group is formed or is discerned to be operating. Up to this point there may be 'group activity', but only when it is recognized and managed can it be said to constitute 'group work'. The structure of your day-release course will influence when this is introduced. It is relatively straightforward in a one-year day-release course for the practice-based registrars to regard the whole year as group work orientated. Group-forming activities will therefore be among the first tasks of the year. Many day-release courses are more complex, with trainees who are simultaneously at different points in the training cycle ('carousel course'). Here priorities have to be evaluated and group considerations tailored accordingly. If the emphasis is on the performance of tasks, a lot of preliminary and management work can be saved by identifying and using subgroups that are already working together.

Carousel groups can function well so long as you are aware of the process issues related to changing membership.

Where the process elements of learning are to be emphasized, a *contract* can specify who does what in the group, what the group does, who the group consists of and how power is exercised and decisions made.

Reluctant or rebellious elements in the group can complicate matters. Although an experienced leader can turn most situations to advantage, any element of coercion is educationally and morally dubious. Both process and task tend to work best with those who are motivated. Any individual must have the right to opt out, although he may be asked to explain why. If the course is heavily group based, special provision may have to be made for that person.

Participants who do not already know each other well, who are at different stages of personal and professional development and who come from a variety of different settings can contribute much to group work, partly by virtue of the 'freshness' of the experience. There is less risk of cliques within the group dominating the scene before the group is established. There is also more potential for enrichment as participants are exposed to many different points of view. On the other hand, groups made up of participants with similar backgrounds, cultures and experiences may work closely together more quickly.

Group work: where?

The context can be an influential element. In a day-release course with one course organizer and one meeting room it is clearly difficult to have more than one identified group. If a motivated minority thinks that they would benefit from a specialized group activity, special provision, such as separate times and venues, will have to be considered.

Postgraduate seminar rooms are usually set up as classrooms, with rows of hard chairs facing a blackboard and lectern. Most group-based activity will involve physically rearranging this set-up, usually to form the chairs into a circle. Whereas a task group may function well in a classroom with all its usual equipment, a process group may perform better in a quiet 'lounge' with comfortable chairs, a minimum of interruptions and relaxed time constraints.

Many courses begin and end each year with residential units. Typically these take place in comfortable hotels or conference centres (although some course organizers advocate group formation through 'roughing it' at an outdoor pursuits centre). The residential setting is very conducive to group work, by providing:

- protected time, free from interruptions (bleeps etc.)
- time out from other ongoing concerns, personal, domestic or work related
- continuous time, unlike the day-release course which is by definition episodic. The availability of a span of days permits a rolling process to operate which generates continuity, momentum and a steeper learning curve
- group-forming opportunities enhanced by the convivial element of working, dining, relaxing and socializing together
- space, comfort and pleasant surroundings
- economy – notwithstanding the high cost of residential modules they can be economical in terms of time, resource persons and materials, and (by permitting specialization of function) protective of expensive day-release course time.

The year-start and year-end residentials can conveniently coincide with group forming and ending tasks. Residentials can be offered at other times for more specialized or targeted purposes.

Group work: how?

'We make our path by walking.' (Community group slogan)

The function of the group leader is vital to the group. Skill in leadership comes from experience, supplemented by going on courses for training in group skills. It does not come from books, although reading can help you organize the learning which takes place in other settings.

Leadership entails two basic functions: task management and holding the boundaries.

Task management

Task management implies preparing and presenting the group task clearly, offering guidelines on how to proceed as the session evolves, and helping the members to remain focused as they work on it. Provision of a suitable environment is basic to this.

Holding the boundaries

This can be compared with the work of a sheepdog or shepherd (although this is not to imply that the members are sheep!). It involves recognizing individual tendencies to break away, taking unobtrusive action to rectify this without causing the 'flock' to stampede or fragment. This shepherding also involves monitoring the group's cohesion, fostering a sense of security and helping it to move as a body along an agreed path.

The group's autonomy deserves recognition since it may exercise choices. After all, there are many ways to achieve a task. The leader monitors the group process and helps it to carry out its tasks.

The leader's best position is on the boundary of the group – somewhat detached and from a vantage point which gives an overview, with an agenda which is not identical to that of the rest of the group but aware of wider issues. This does not imply non-participation or dominance but a watchful and supportive involvement. From the boundary, the leader can make suggestions, identify problems and orchestrate corrective action, take a longer view of crises as they occur, give feedback, and identify and deal with unfinished business.

Exercising leadership in small group work requires an understanding of group dynamics, and is described further in that context in Chapter 11.

Exercise 16

(a) Extend this list of ways in which the trainee benefits from working in a group at the day-release course.

1 Social
2 Group support of peers
3
4
5
6

(b) In what sense does each of these require the presence of the other participants?

For example:
collaboration
affirmation
information
confrontation

Scenario: A further discussion between Dr Meeke and Dr Best

Meeke: *Groups – I've had it up to here with groups! I've always had a fairly open mind about these things. I've been to a few trainers' courses where there was some group stuff, but this is different.*

Best: *What's the difference?*

Meeke: *The difference is that we behaved ourselves in groups and tried to get something done. In fact, once we behaved ourselves so well that the organizer got up-tight about it and tried to cause arguments. But this lot, they don't know how to behave in a group – it's a disaster! I'm thinking of going back to talks on ECGs and liver function and things like that, given by consultants. At least the trainees would think they were doing something useful.*

Best: *Why do you think they'd prefer that?*

Meeke: *It's familiar, for a start. They would know where they are at – so would the consultants and so would I. I suppose you would call that collusion.*

Best: *So why not collude if it makes everybody happy?*

Meeke: *It's not good enough in the long run. One of my ideas for the course is to make the best use of the time when the trainees come together. That means leaving aside things they can get from books, things they mostly already know and things they can get through their trainer, one-to-one.*

Best: *Which brings you back to... ?*

Meeke: *Group work. Yes I know. But it's not working. Everyone arrives at different times, the SHOs are always dashing out to answer their bleep, someone's always on call that night and has to leave before we're finished, some look bored, others won't shut up. And they always want to talk about something else. One doesn't show up to group-type sessions. When I tackled him on that he said he had done something else because there didn't seem to be much on the programme that day. It's depressing! Yesterday, one actually accused another of malpractice. Nearly led to a walkout.*

Best: *It seems to me that you've been to a few group courses and the trainees haven't. You know how you behave in a group and they don't behave the same way. Can you pinpoint where the problem lies?*

Meeke: *I suppose it must be something to do with me. How should they know what to do about group work? It's not something they've been into before, after all; and I am the course organizer. What would you do?*

Best: *You seem to have strong feelings about this group, tell me about them.*

Meeke: *I hate this group. No... I'm angry with them... I feel a failure. Hey, you're beginning to sound like a social worker. What does it matter what I feel about it? Everybody says you have to do group work. So it's got to be done, and I'm beginning to hate those sessions. Maybe I should get somebody else to do the groupie bits. Maybe I should just let somebody else take over the whole lot and go back to being a GP. At least with one patient at a time I know what I'm doing.*

Best: *I think you're saying two things. First, your honeymoon period is over and you're getting to grips with real problems. The second is called cognitive dissonance – I know, more jargon. There's a conflict between your expectations and the reality as you perceive it. Maybe the people in the group are feeling it too. You might raise that for discussion. When both parties to a transaction experience and work on their dissonance, change is likely to happen. That's not just learning, that's growth. Attitudes change, a new situation arises. You're right about one thing – as course organizer, changes start with you. So I have two suggestions.*

       Don't run away from the discomfort you're feeling, learn to recognize it. It's a signpost, a turning point, a crisis in the technical sense, if you like. And it's as relevant to patient management in the practice as it is to leading the trainee group. The other thing is to take up the issues it raises. What is group work? What is its place in the course, if any? In what respects is the group malfunctioning? And what does this tell you about how the group should be helped?

Meeke: *But that could take ages. It could mean reading books and going on courses. What about next week?*

Best: *Plan your approach for the shorter and longer term. Chase up books and courses by all means. Meanwhile, have a look at a few articles – the ACO Journal is a good place to start.*

Meeke: *What journal?*

Best: *Ah – it's got a different name now – Education for General Practice. Here's a small book you can borrow too – it's all cartoons and one-liners. Once upon a group, it's called.*

Meeke: *Okay, but what about next week?*

Best: *You're really putting me on the spot. Like any GP I know that giving advice rarely works. But I'm getting old enough now to break the rules. So one simple piece of advice for next week. Instead of getting up-tight when something goes wrong, just tell the group how you're feeling. I bet that'll stir things up a bit!*

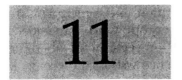

Group dynamics

Introduction

If the preceding chapter explored the anatomy of the group, this chapter examines the physiology and pathology. To carry the analogy further, group leadership training is the therapeutics part of the curriculum. There are some natural group leaders, but most of us have to study group dynamics and practise the leadership role.

The developmental model

Tuckman (1965) described group dynamics in terms of a developmental life cycle with four phases: forming, storming, norming and performing. In physiological terms it seems rational that we should consider adding a fifth one: ending. Tuckman's model provides a framework for understanding apparently irrational behaviour within the group. A summary of his stages is shown in Figure 11.1. The ending phase recalls the Kübler-Ross model of grief. All of the phases relate to the overall life cycle of the group, but may manifest themselves in minor ways in the dynamics of an individual group session.

Awareness of this scheme will help you to diagnose difficulties within the group, whether a problem is purely developmental, i.e. part of the physiology, or a disorder which threatens the group, i.e. pathology. If a leader overreacts to a physiological event in the group and rushes to extinguish it, he may be creating a pathological situation.

The developmental model suggests that there is a group identity. This competes with each participant's individual identity and may give rise to behaviour within the group which is at odds with the normal behaviour of the individuals. It is reminiscent of Balint's 'collusion of anonymity' and 'dilution of responsibility'. Things can be blamed on the group if individual identity (and therefore responsibility) is suspended. Patterns of mutual inhibition or synergism between group members may appear alarming. In pharmacology the phenomena of drug inhibition and synergism are related to receptor sites. The equivalent of the receptor site in group work is the 'locus of control' – the leader, the usurper of leadership, the attention-seeking member, the comedian – all putting in bids for their own form of influence within the group. If events are seen as the result of interaction at such loci of control, corrective interventions can be undertaken. Group roles such as usurper, comedian and scapegoat are considered later in this chapter.

How to lead the group

The main tasks of the leader during the life span of a group are considered under the following headings: getting started, climate building, leadership behaviour, nurturing the group, coping with difficult members, giving feedback, evaluation and closing the session.

Getting started

Baggage dump is a useful term for the initial phase of a group session. Members arrive in various stages of preparedness, feeling rushed and preoccupied with the previous events or plans for later. They may need to deal with these preoccupations before they can focus on the work of the group. Making the transition from the outer world to the world of the group may mean letting off steam. Briefly sharing such preoccupations is helpful, perhaps with a symbolic exercise such as 'write down what is on your mind and put it in the waste paper basket; you may reclaim it afterwards if you wish'.

The attitude of the group leader will set the tone initially. If he is purposeful, businesslike and practical this will be communicated to the group members and they are likely to mirror his behaviour. This is *'modelling'*.

Establish or rehearse the understandings upon which the group functions. These rules should be made by the members of the group and explicitly agreed. Once they are established they need to be alluded to only briefly at the start of each session. If the group 'owns' its rules, the members are likely to respect them. It is a matter of agreement as to who will enforce them – the leader or the group as a whole. The list of rules may include such items as:

- confidentiality – there are degrees of confidentiality and it is seldom absolute. A basic agreement should ensure that the personal statements of individuals will be respected and not quoted outside the group
- punctuality – to minimize disruption and facilitate the group tasks

1 *Forming*
Defining the nature and boundaries of the task:
- grumbling about the task or setting
- meandering, ineffective approach to the task
- showing suspicion of the task, and each other
- testing the leader, and each other
- approaching the task with hesitation or avoidance behaviour

2 *Storming*
Questioning the value of the exercise:
- challenging the leader, and each other
- experimenting with hostility, aggression and frustration
- defensively resisting self-disclosure
- showing rivalry, argument, rebellion and opposition

3 *Norming*
Opening up and inviting each other to:
- express feelings
- re-define the task
- give and take opinions, evaluate them
- feel like a group
- offer mutual support and build special relationships
- clarify leadership and show more unity and consensus
- show more cohesion and group feeling, less interest in extrinsic factors

4 *Performing*
Pursuing the task effectively by:
- contributing frequently and mutually
- showing more insight and understanding of the task
- not worrying about interpersonal issues (which should have been sorted or relegated)
- feeling safe and confident of the identity and task of the group
- gaining real achievements

5 *Ending*
Facing the loss of the group experience:
- by denying it – 'we'll meet again...'
- by bargaining – 'our task is not yet complete...'
- with anger – 'nobody appreciates what we have achieved...'
- with depression – 'parting is such sweet sorrow'
- with a sense of ritual – 'bury it decently and move on'

Figure 11.1 The developmental model (after Tuckman, 1965).

- fixed starting and ending times – most people don't like marathons but will support an agreed decision
- leadership – the group may exercise leadership functions, which may be devolved or circulated even in the presence of an overall leader
- the ownership of statements – they should not be attributed outside the group, i.e. not 'some people say that...' but 'I feel that...'.

Agreeing rules and task setting are part of *contract forming*.

The leader or a member of the group introduces the group task and explains it carefully so that it is understood and agreed. Much of the work for this may have to be done in advance by the leader in terms of teaching/learning objectives, preferably written. This facilitates the later task of evaluation. A statement of such tasks may take the following form.

1 Briefly describe the task to be carried out, e.g. prepare and perform a role-play advising a diabetic patient about nutrition.
2 What do I wish the group to learn?
3 Are there additional objectives, e.g. enjoyment?
4 Are there objectives related to individuals, e.g. to the quiet one?
5 Do I have objectives for me, e.g. to practise my use of time?
6 What would indicate success in each of these?

The mature group may wish to take responsibility for its own task setting.

Climate building

Openness and confidence spring from a sense of security in the group. Modelling on the leader is an important starting point; his verbal and non-verbal behaviour contribute to the real work of helping members to participate as fully as possible. Knowing that the leader is not 'shockable', judgemental or fearful enables the others to overcome their own tendencies in these directions.

Participation can be invited, not coerced. Icebreakers are helpful here. Even then it may be necessary to foster participation by directing remarks and questions, eliciting statements or even using silence constructively. Differences in levels of participation should be accepted and perhaps discussed.

It is also important to maintain a balance between task orientation and humour. The group comedian may be useful for breaking the ice, but he can soon become a liability. Care must be taken that no one feels he is the butt of a joke. Again, modelling is important here.

The aim is to function co-operatively; the group is not about some members 'winning' and others 'losing'. Competitiveness may be helpful if there is more than one subgroup working on the same task, but it is disruptive as a force within the group. If it exists, it should be discussed openly.

Time should be found at the end of each session to see whether there are unresolved issues in any of these areas. If the leader senses that a group member has been
hurt, it may be necessary to discuss this with the individual outside the group.

Leadership behaviour

Much behaviour in the group will result from modelling on the leader, especially the
more intangible qualities like attitudes, genuineness and integrity. Doctors as group
leaders are often less democratic than they might be because of their own earlier
educational experiences. The good leader exhibits a number of basic qualities:

- encouraging the group to identify and solve its own problems
- encouraging the quiet ones and enabling the more dominant to take a back seat
- recognizing crises, e.g. bids for leadership, formation of pairs/sub-groups, opting
  out behaviour, and bringing them into the open for discussion and resolution
- being aware of defences, thus creating an atmosphere where they can be lowered
- promoting the autonomy of the group
- caring for the members of the group without creating dependence
- intervening to protect the scapegoat, moderating the giving of feedback and
  rescuing any 'group casualties'
- giving some insight into what is happening
- having 'befores' and 'afters', i.e. preparation and follow-up, to protect the time and
  energy of the group and foster its ability to achieve its tasks
- taking the longer view and remaining calm in the face of conflict, leadership bids,
  silence or criticism.

Nurturing the group

From this semi-detached position the leader watches the process, the task and the
individuals as they interact. He is aware of the aims (his own and those of the group),
and the need to evaluate, summarize, identify unfinished business and keep time. He
respects the dignity and individuality of the members while fostering the autonomy
of the group. He is sensitive to changes in atmosphere, viewing them in developmental (see the life cycle of the group) and dynamic terms. He actively facilitates while
being as non-directive as possible. He protects the vulnerabilities of the members. He
regards crises as opportunities for learning and teaching. He does not avoid conflict,
but utilizes the resources of the group to discuss problems, find productive resolu-
tions and promote insight. He is able to identify and deal with the feelings generated
in himself through the exercise in ways (and at times) which do not interfere with
the group process or the fulfilment of the task. His main enemies in the group are

boredom, loss of participation and his own needs for recognition and approval in the short term.

All this may seem a bit daunting, but the list is reminiscent of the Leeuwenhorst definition of the GP and these activities are the group equivalent of consultation tasks and skills in the surgery. There are no perfect group leaders, just as there are no perfect GPs, but learning can take place and performance can improve with practice.

Coping with difficult members

Every course organizer fears having 'difficult' group members such as the extreme attention-seeker. One cannot expect to love every one of them all the time, and the 'collusion of cosiness' is a very flawed strategy.

A well-functioning group is a potent instrument of change. Change should not be forced, but it can be facilitated. The danger of scapegoating must be borne in mind. Acceptance of group norms and feedback within the group usually curb deviant behaviour while maintaining respect for individuality.

People in groups exhibit problem behaviour for a variety of reasons. Some are due to personality factors. Group relationships are complex; when eight people interact in a group there are 28 one-to-one relationships, and there are bound to be conflicts. The aim is not group therapy (and certainly not psychotherapy). It pays to have realistic goals.

If group members are difficult, it is generally because they are sceptical, silent, dominant (too talkative), bored, withdrawn, aggressive, reluctant to attend, flippant, clowning, inarticulate, shy, distracting, attention seeking or vulnerable. The resources of the group can be employed to discuss or confront behaviour which is disruptive to the group. The method employed should be in line with Pendleton's rules. Positive statements should come first, then any criticism should take the form of recommendations for change. In the words of the hymn, one should 'guard each man's dignity and save each man's pride...' (with apologies to the women!).

One of the limiting factors in group work is the autonomy of the group. This is a fundamental precept akin to the autonomy of the patient in clinical practice. It is there to protect the group from exploitation and manipulation by the leader and permits members to exercise informed consent. Only with consent can a group move from the safe waters of task orientation to the more personally challenging high seas of process or 'growth' work. Although much useful work can be achieved through task orientation it is through process orientation that participants learn about themselves, their attitudes, prejudices and hidden agendas, and gain insight and skills in 'person management'.

Respect for the group's autonomy is equally important as a protection for the leader. It is impossible to escape a sense of frustration or failure when one's legitimate aims are not achieved. Leaders do not have the right to coerce the group – this is self-defeating. If challenges are not well received by the group the issues should be discussed by the group and, if necessary, left aside. Unfortunately, it only takes one dissenter to block movement. Like the wartime convoy the group may have to move at a pace dictated by the least agile members and zigzag to avoid threats and dangers. The leader can facilitate but not guarantee progress. This is the responsibility of the group as a whole, and not the undiluted success or failure of leadership.

Difficult behaviour by members which operates at the task level is usually easily addressed by redefining the task and discussing behaviour which impedes it, brainstorming, problem solving and simple confrontation. Tuckman's model is useful as a diagnostic aid.

Process orientation unveils problems among participants of a different order. Those whose cognitive style is inherently hostile to interactions which are perceived as embarrassing or intrusive are liable to become obstructive. Where this takes the form of withdrawal behind defences the group may still be able to function, respecting the person's autonomy by making allowance for a form of 'observer status'. Occasionally there are manifestations of rebellion, anger or hostility. Where this is limited consistently to one person he or she will merit special attention from the leader – invited to make a statement, voluntarily withdraw from such activities, or discuss one-to-one outside the group setting. In such circumstances the leader must adopt an open, calm, non-threatening approach. Frontal assaults on highly defended positions in a group setting might accomplish something but there will be casualties on both sides.

Seating arrangements may have significant influence. Individuals who are colluding together may need to be separated. One who needs protection can be placed close to the leader. The attention-seeker may be moved to a position where he does not so readily catch the leader's eye.

Giving feedback

Most people's experience of receiving feedback in everyday life tends to be negative. Group work provides a unique opportunity to get feedback in a positive, caring environment from colleagues whose opinions are respected. Feedback is part of group membership. It happens whether we want it or not. If it is not deliberate and constructive there will be a vacuum which will be filled with non-verbal and unintentional messages, and it will be subject to misinterpretation. Feedback plays an essential role in organizing the learning which is taking place and should be an integral part of group work. It functions at several levels.

1 To the individual: from the leader and from peers. Properly monitored and exercised, this can be a potent tool for change and growth.
2 To the group: from the leader and from members. This addresses process, task and evaluation issues.

3 To the leader: from the group and from individuals. This may contribute towards evaluation of aspects of the course.

Feedback should be compassionate, professional and reciprocal, in order to protect the group from the abuse of the power gap. When individuals are giving feedback to their peers there should be a particular purpose, i.e. random feedback should be discouraged, and controls (to avoid disasters like scapegoating).

All such situations should be regulated since it is feedback that makes groups and individuals most vulnerable. It is important for group members to learn the necessary skills and values. This is best imparted by modelling on the leader along the following suggested lines (Hopson and Scally, 1981):

- feedback should be offered, not imposed
- it should be descriptive rather than evaluative
- it should be specific and should refer to features or behaviours that can be changed
- it should emphasize positives rather than negatives
- if negative, it should include a positive suggestion
- the person giving feedback should take responsibility for it
- the feedback should be checked with others.

This process gives individuals a lot of information about themselves and how to achieve what they want within a protected and supportive environment. These rules are fundamental to group work. They are the group equivalent of the counselling tradition of Karl Rogers which allows people to reflect, gain insight, grow and change in a supportive atmosphere.

Evaluation

This is an important aspect of any educational exercise. The group should be responsible for evaluating its own performance at two levels.

1 Self-assessment by each individual, based on questions such as:
   - what did I like about the way I worked in this session?
   - what might I wish to change next time I do it?
   - what was the most memorable thing about this session?
2 An examination of overall aims and tasks achieved by the group, reflecting on what made the group effective or what hindered its pursuit of the task, and what might have been done differently.

Participants may find it difficult to accept that the group leader is also a judge of their individual behaviour. Evaluating the effectiveness of the group is certainly a proper concern for the course organizer, but assessment of members' performance will complicate process issues and is probably better carried out in other ways. Clearly the course organizer will get to know his trainees in some depth through participation in group work, and this will facilitate the formative aspects of the assessment activities applied within the course.

Closing the session

As in drama, a good finale can rescue even a mediocre performance. The main tasks are to finish as close as possible to the agreed time while leaving time for the 'house-keeping' aspects of the session. The group should not be allowed to disintegrate (with members leaving piecemeal), drag on (to exhaustion/frustration limits) or end precipitately (with no provision for dealing with evaluation and loose ends). Ending often takes more time than anticipated. It is therefore important that the group is time conscious throughout and that there should be some kind of countdown towards the end, helping to focus the group progressively on its objectives.

A final checklist might include elements such as:

1 Summarizing:
   • what has been learned, gained and achieved – this can be done in the whole group or in pairs (with feedback to the group)
   • what we did (task fulfilment)
   • how we did it (process).
2 Following up (action required, tasks delegated) and planning the next session (preparation, tasks delegated).
3 Dealing with unfinished business:
   • identifying issues and feelings and agreeing how and when to deal with them
   • being aware of unresolved feelings, conflicts and dilemmas
   • de-roling – focus the group on the present – and returning to everyday concerns so that the group concerns are not carried forward beyond the end of the session.
4 Closing on a positive note.

Tool-kit

In undertaking group work, the leader needs a tool-kit of activities which may be drawn upon as the need arises. This tool-kit should be expanded constantly. The proper use of tools takes practice. There are many books of games and exercises for group activities (*see* Part 6). The following is merely an attempt to classify them with brief examples.

1 *Icebreakers:* These are introductory activities for making the transition from the world without to the inner world of the group. For example:
   • naming each other round the circle
   • introducing each other in pairs
   • 'party games'.

2 *Orientation exercises* such as:
- sharing in pairs what has happened since last meeting
- off-loading burdensome 'luggage'. Each person comes with his own preoccupations. Get rid of these by talking them through or dumping them symbolically on the sidelines.

3 *Listening exercises*: These involve getting in pairs and taking turns to talk and listen about matters of individual concern. The listening party should remain silent. A similar exercise involves 'trios', a speaker, a listener and an observer who notes the process issues. The roles then rotate.

4 *Exploratory exercises:*
- truthful personal statements are written down, randomized and 'picked out of the hat'. Then each person, in turn, presents and defends the statement he has picked out as if it were his own
- paired sharing on specific questions, e.g. things that make me angry or anxious
- individuals taking turns to address the group on such themes as 'what I hope to get from this group'
- group members are asked to sort themselves along a notional line on the basis of a variety of qualities, e.g. leadership or influence within the group, participation level, comfort with group work etc. The distribution is discussed and analysed. They may then be invited to rearrange themselves in the light of the discussion. A further 'twist' is to ask them to place each other along the line and comment on the decisions made. This provides a non-threatening form of feedback.

5 *Growth exercises:*
- hot-seat: volunteers invite feedback from the group in a structured setting
- fishbowl: two or more members are observed by the rest, carrying out a task such as discussion or role-play with feedback
- carousel: place chairs in two concentric circles, facing each other in pairs. Provocative questions/statements/role-play scenarios are allocated to each member of the inner circle. At intervals the outer circle rotates by one place so that each participant is exposed to a different challenge every few minutes. Then the positions are reversed.

6 *Group task exercises*, with the group process observer, include:
- producing a plan, project, protocol or case discussion
- problem solving, e.g. the 'survival in the desert' game where the group has to negotiate priorities and decisions in a simulated crisis.

7 *Ending exercises*, in sub-groups or all together, may involve discussion with feedback under headings such as:
- summarizing
- what happened for me during this session
- planning the next meeting
- what I am looking forward to after this session
- retrieving the 'luggage' from the shelf (the reverse of baggage dump).

The course organizer's safety net

This part began by acknowledging the apprehensions with which most of us approach group leading. These pages may even have heightened the discomfort. Reference has been made to the similarity between leading and managing the consultation. As GPs we all started with a simple approach to our consultations, limited aims and a good deal of trepidation. We also experienced the value of being able to discuss problems with a colleague – a senior partner or a trainer. The same should apply to the early stages of learning how to work with a group of trainees. Many schemes employ the services of group-work facilitators. This is not opting out. Apprenticeship is a good way to learn.

If you are not able to do this, you may have a steeper learning curve. The imagination allows no limit to the number of things that can go wrong. In reality, if you start with limited aims and simple tasks, you will soon begin to reap the rewards. The dangers are mostly to yourself. As group leader you may be left holding the residue of the group's unfinished business. Experienced group leaders know the value of having a personal 'therapist' with whom to work through any unresolved feelings which it is not appropriate to share with the group (as Dr Meeke does with Dr Best). Find yourself a mentor whose discretion and support you can rely on.

Summary

1 Group work is an integral part of the day-release course.
2 The course organizer is the *de facto* leader.
3 He learns group work by doing it, by attending group training courses, and to some extent by reading about it.
4 He should have a mentor with whom he can 'let off steam' or discuss problems.
5 There should be a purpose for the group work and a desire to explore the potential of the group for growth.
6 The least threatening group work is task centred.
7 The group task is the overt agenda at a given time.
8 The group process is everything which goes on in the group as it pursues its task.
9 There is no group task without process.
10 If the task is undefined, process takes over.
11 A group should not be doing process-orientated work without an experienced leader.
12 The purpose of the group should be defined, agreed and evaluated.
13 The group should be encouraged to identify its own needs and solve its own problems – otherwise it is a class.

14 The more 'befores' and 'afters' with the group, the better the educational experience will be.

15 Ground rules must be agreed in advance and enforced by the group.

16 My rules are about:
- punctuality and time keeping
- participation (how to deal with opting out)
- confidentiality – degrees of absolute
- owned statement ('I think...' not 'some people think...')
- direct address – person-to-person (I – you)
- who will enforce the rules?
- applying Pendleton's rules – positive first; criticism must be constructive and positive.

17 Group leadership involves managing the whole group experience with sensitivity and insight

18 The tasks of the leader are:
- getting started
- climate building
- facilitating
- modelling desired behaviour
- observing process, task and time
- coping with difficult situations/members
- feedback, evaluation
- closing.

19 Have fun, make it fun!

Further reading on groups

Group dynamics, process and experiential learning

Heron J (1989) *The facilitator's handbook*. Kogan Page, London. (Contains a model for analysis of group facilitation and discusses the main options open to facilitators in any kind of experiential learning group.)

Hopson B and Scally M (1981) *Life skills teaching*. McGraw-Hill, London. (Discusses the use of group work in schools and gives general group-work guidelines.)

Houston G (1990) *Red book of groups*. The Rochester Foundation, 8 Rochester Terrace, London. (To help facilitation skills – a classic booklet on group leading.)

Johnson D *et al.* (1991) *Joining together*. Prentice-Hall, London.

Kindred M (1987) *Once upon a group ...* Privately published, 20 Dover Street, Southwell, Nottingham NG25 0EZ. (Cartoons and one-liners; a witty, clear guide to dos and don'ts.)

Pfeiffer JW and Jones JE (1983) *The handbook of structured experiences for human relations training.* University Associates, US. (Guidelines for group leaders on an experiential approach to learning.)

Tuckman BW (1965) Developmental sequences in small groups. *Psychological Bulletin,* **63**: 384–99. (Forming, norming, storming, performing etc.)

Group exercises and games

Brandes D and Phillips H (1990) *The gamester's handbook. Games for teachers and group workers.* Hutchinson, London.

Brandes D (1990) *The gamester's handbook II. More games for teachers and group workers.* Hutchinson, London.

Brandreth G (1981) *Everyman's indoor games.* Dent, London.

Johnstone M (1987) *Children's party games.* Ward Lock, London.

Kindred M and Kindred M (1998) *Once upon a group: exercises.* 4M Publications, Southwell, Notts.

Groups for personal growth

Egan G (1976) *Interpersonal living. Skills/contract approach to interpersonal growth training in groups.* Brooks Cole Publishing Co., USA.

Smith PB (1980) *Small groups and personal growth.* Methuen, London.

There have also been many useful articles in: *Education for General Practice,* the *Journal of the Association of Course Organizers* and *Horizons.*

Part 4

The SHO years

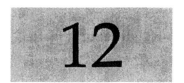

The hospital contribution to vocational training

Introduction

'There is much that a doctor in training can gain from experience as a hospital SHO.' (RCGP, 1994a)

The senior house officer (SHO) has tended to be the second-class citizen of vocational training. The focus of vocational training, and its resources, has been mainly on the practice trainee (registrar). SHOs are in a double bind: the regulations require an extensive period of hospital training in service posts, indicating that they are hospital doctors; the vocational training scheme, however, tells them they are vocational trainees for general practice, without necessarily ensuring that the hospitals make appropriate provision.

The course organizer also experiences this dilemma. He is expected to provide a meaningful educational programme both for SHOs and for registrars. However, it is difficult to identify who the relevant SHOs are and to integrate their erratic attendance with the continuity required for group learning by the registrars.

Much effort has been invested throughout the 1990s by all interested parties to address and redress dissonances arising from the hospital component. The outcome is a growing literature and a healthy debate.

The role of the course organizer

Course organizers undertake a variety of tasks in relation to SHOs:

- providing the day-release course programme and helping with regional provision, giving advice, support and counselling for career and personal problems

- representing the regional director locally and briefing him on local issues
- liaising with hospital postgraduate tutors and consultants on educational matters
- helping with the filling and monitoring of approved posts
- advising hospitals about approved posts and packages
- shortlisting and interviewing prospective SHOs, along with hospital tutors
- helping with the assessment of SHO trainees in post
- attending the hospital education committee
- trouble-shooting when problems arise with SHOs and posts
- encouraging local initiatives as they arise.

Not all course organizers perform all of these duties. There is no simple, overall pattern because no one is in overall command of training for SHOs. The course organizer has no powers or statutory function and his responsibilities are, therefore, undefined.

Theme and variations: variables

Each scheme experiences problems specific to its own circumstances. The variables include:

- the number of course organizers: single (dispersed) or small teams (centralized)
- the number and variety of hospitals and how they relate to the educational facility for the day-release course (usually a hospital postgraduate centre); distance and lines of communication
- the number of SHOs, either on self-constructed schemes (who are difficult to identify) or on rotational packages
- the local consultants in charge of approved SHO posts: their awareness of GP educational issues and their commitment to the educational process
- the hospitals' policies about protected time for learning: 'in-house', half-day release and study leave
- the regional guidelines and provision for SHO training.

Theme and variations: problems

Problems specific to the SHO trainee

These lie mainly in the areas of identity, conditions and morale. Problems of identity stem from:

- an unstructured and unformed relationship with general practice

- lack of knowledge about how to prepare for general practice while in hospital. Kearley (1990) quoted one SHO as saying: *'I don't really know what GPs actually do – I've only ever done hospital stuff'*
- being uninformed about GP issues and having little contact with real GPs
- being in a transitional state and having divided loyalties
- 'hospital collusion' or medical ethos (Tait, 1987) – the explicit or implicit belief sustained among hospital doctors, irrespective of grade, which assumes the primacy of institutional, disease-centred perspectives over the community and patient-centred perspective of general practice. Kearley quoted another typical observation: *'General practitioners were never involved as teachers within the hospital'*
- identification with the hospital setting through years of formation, and with hospital peers through intense interaction
- potential dropout from 'real medicine' – second-class hospital doctor.

Problems relating to conditions include:

- heavy workload and service commitment leading to fatigue and stress
- the lack of continuity caused by having a new job, new boss and, perhaps, a new home every six months
- the fact that educational provision may take low priority, especially when hospitals are undergoing cutbacks and change in management structure and staffing levels
- difficulties in getting leave for study and day-release courses because of ignorance of the entitlements, problems of 'cover', peer pressure, non-co-operation by the institution and lack of direction
- poor living quarters, catering and amenities.

Morale may be affected adversely as a consequence of:

- problems of identity and conditions
- contractual changes and the feeling that general practice is being used as a political football
- prospects or realities of medical unemployment
- professional, personal and family demands at a vulnerable stage of life
- the feeling that life is passing them by while they work.

Many of these factors are shared by all SHOs. However, there seems to be a pattern emerging among GP trainees which results in the resolve to 'get away from it all' as soon as they can, for a while at least. They may drop out at this stage; others continue into the practice year, but do not proceed to take up full-time practice posts, preferring to work part-time or take up salaried options. This is contributing to the 'recruitment crisis' within general practice.

Problems for the hospital

For training purposes the hospital does not manage positively the distinction between the needs of SHOs intending to specialize in hospital medicine and those who are oriented towards general practice. At best it treats them all as mini-specialists. Its departmental structure is not well suited to generalist and interdisciplinary training. Hospital specialists generally have poorly formed views concerning educational priorities for GP training (RCGP, 1988). They are not well equipped for their teaching task and may lack formal training in educational skills. This is being addressed through the formation of hospital education committees, partly as a result of heightened awareness of educational values on the part of the specialty colleges.

Hospitals are run on SHO power. Whatever emphasis is accorded to the training function of the grade, service considerations come first – frequently at the expense of all other factors. Posts have to be filled, and unpopular posts are often inserted into general practice training rotations. There is a high turnover of SHOs. Unless organized as rotational programmes it is difficult for hospital teachers to keep track of the needs, welfare and progress of the individual SHO.

Protected time for learning is difficult to reconcile with the service demand. There are criteria concerning learning time, but institutional considerations predominate. Study leave is easiest to administer in blocks, and half-day release is seen as disruptive and of low priority. Authorities are more sympathetic to requests to devote study leave to specialist diplomas, whether or not these are of educative value.

The visitations by specialist colleges to approve posts increasingly involve nominees of the RCGP as full voting members. These visits are influential but episodic, external inspections. This top-down approach cannot generate an internal momentum for reform.

Problems for the course organizer

These factors in turn lead to specific problems for the course organizer because:

- erratic attendance by SHO trainees is subversive to the half-day release programme
- educational aims and values tend towards the lowest common denominator
- the continuity required by an evolving, group-based programme is disrupted
- SHOs come to the course with the sort of expectations fostered by the hospital. Frequently they value the didactic and are impatient with 'soft' knowledge
- enlisting the co-operation of the hospitals and their consultants can be very time consuming
- in selecting SHOs there is often a conflict of values between the course organizer and consultants on the interviewing panel (they select for a good SHO; the course organizer selects for GP potential)

- getting to know the shifting population of SHO trainees is difficult
- when the release course serves a number of hospitals, lines of communication are stretched
- administrative back-up in the task is frequently basic
- the course organizer's role is ill defined in relation to hospitals, and he may therefore lack credibility.

Theme and variations: responses

National, regional and local initiatives have resulted in a variety of responses to this varied picture.

1 SCOPME (1991) has issued a useful report on the situation of all SHOs.
2 The RCGP in 1993 published outline educational objectives in paediatrics, geriatrics, obstetrics and gynaecology, accident and emergency medicine, palliative medicine and psychiatry in conjunction with the respective colleges and a statement on the quality of hospital-based education for general practice (RCGP, 1993).
3 Regions, in conjunction with the JCPTGP, are gaining greater GP influence over the visits of the specialty colleges to hospital posts for approval and reapproval.
4 RCGP faculties and regional postgraduate councils are fostering dialogue between GP and hospital teachers on educational issues.
5 The British Medical Association has issued a document outlining study leave provision (GMSC, 1996). This is summarized in Chapter 16.

Other initiatives are beginning to redress the problems of identity and conditions for SHO trainees, for example:

- the provision of sandwich courses (an initial period in a training practice before undertaking general hospital training)
- expansion of the practice-based element of vocational training to 18 months, and reducing the hospital element to 18 months (as in the armed services and parts of Scotland) is being proposed as the norm from 1998
- separation of day-release courses for SHOs and registrars
- abandoning day-release courses for SHOs in favour of residential teaching blocks
- attachment to a GP mentor/tutor throughout the hospital years for periodic tutorial and surgery visits
- exploitation of all the facilities of the hospital for interdisciplinary education and instruction in information technology, library skills and audit work
- in the Republic of Ireland SHOs' study leave is ear-marked for exam purposes and a week of job experience in a training practice during each six-month post. The half-day release course is *additional* protected time.

The course organizer can help by:

- making a real effort to identify SHO trainees, and meeting them to explore the educational potential of their individual situations
- trying to adapt the day-release course to their needs and making it easy for them to attend, without sacrificing the value for registrars (who may act as useful mentors for SHOs on an individual basis)
- working the common ground. The hospital needs the SHO trainees to fill its posts. You need the hospital and its staff on your side to create a situation where SHO trainees both receive an educational experience of worth and obtain release from ward duties to attend the day-release course. There can be a convergence of interests
- bringing GP education *into the hospital* for the benefit of all, including consultants, if the SHOs cannot get leave *from* the hospital for day-release course. Speaking at interdisciplinary or ward meetings, or running joint meetings with the clinical tutor, will establish you as a presence in the hospital territory
- liaising with key consultants about the content of training and methods of formative assessment. There are opportunities for communication through the hospital clinical tutor or chairman of the medical staff committee (or equivalent). Role reversal goes down badly – try telling consultants what they ought to be doing and see how far you get!
- where there is more than one course organizer each can monitor the educational content of a few key posts. Regular meetings are good for SHO morale and maintain the consultants' awareness of their needs
- involving consultants in teaching on the day-release course in accordance with *your* educational principles. They should be briefed tactfully and specifically beforehand
- helping the hospital with the selection and induction of new SHOs and using this as an opportunity to discuss study leave and other vocational training issues
- trying to put educational audit on the agenda of the hospital audit committee
- forging links between individual SHOs and GP trainers, and using the trainers' workshop to brainstorm on local possibilities
- keeping SHO issues on the agenda of the regional postgraduate council's general practice committee
- keeping the regional director informed of problems; there are sanctions which can be invoked through the postgraduate council, Joint Committee and college visitors
- not giving up. Things are changing and improvement in the SHO component is a substantial growth area in vocational training. As the Latin grammar might say: past imperfect, present tense, future perfect.

Present tense, future perfect

'Most consultants have no direct experience of general practice and hence find it difficult to help GP trainees to appreciate the relevance of their hospital experience to their future work as GPs.' (RCGP, 1988)

It is estimated that between 40 and 50% of all SHOs are destined for general practice (RCGP, 1994a; RCP, 1997). Who is responsible for their educational development – the SHOs themselves, the hospital trusts, the consultants, the postgraduate Dean, the regional directors, the respective Royal Colleges, the Joint Committee? All are fiercely independent entities. The lines of communication are complex, perhaps tangled. Does this let the course organizer off the hook? It recalls Balint's concepts of the 'dilution of responsibility' and 'collusion of anonymity'. Perhaps this is why progress for SHOs comes late in the history of vocational training in the UK. A national conference on the needs of SHOs adopted the title *The Lost Tribes* (Dillner, 1993).

The late 1980s produced evidence from many directions of growing unease about the state of SHO training in general. The SCOPME (1991) report *Improving the experience* was a turning point, addressing all aspects of the problem – the workload, living conditions and educational provision. This has been taken up by all the main stakeholders resulting in a tide of contributions covering areas such as:

- the views of junior doctors (Kearley, 1990; Dillner 1993; Torry, 1996)
- the relationship between consultants and course organizers (Styles *et al.*, 1993)
- the contribution of general practitioners to hospital visits (Hand, 1994)
- the balance between hospital- and practice-based training (Calman, 1995)
- the learning curriculum for general practice training in hospitals (the RCGP series of booklets defining, in collaboration with sister colleges, the learning content of SHO posts).

The Calman Report (Calman, 1993) is among the most radical official documents on medical training in recent years. Its purpose was to implement the EU directives on specialist training and plan for their implications. A supplementary report (Calman, 1995) considered the implications for general practice training. Among the recommendations were:

- more co-operation between general practice and hospital teachers
- improved training for all SHOs
- review of selection of hospital posts
- training for general practice to be regarded as equivalent to basic specialist training
- greater flexibility in training, notably to vary the duration of hospital posts for vocational training
- hospital career trainees should benefit from experience in general practice.

These recommendations have fundamental significance. They make possible an 'exchange of hostages' between training practices and hospitals and remove the basis for regarding general practice as an inferior calling. They also allow for the expansion of practice-based training with shorter, more flexible hospital attachment related to the specific needs of individual trainees.

The RCGP policy document *Education and training for general practice* (RCGP, 1994b) acknowledged the prevalence of criticism of hospital-based training but added an interpretation that 'insufficient advantage is being taken of the learning opportunities afforded by hospital posts'.

An excellent report by the Royal College of Physicians (RCP, 1997) takes this point further by defining among other things a core curriculum of generic skills appropriate to SHOs in all hospital posts. If implemented, this, along with their recommendations about teaching, supervision and appraisal, will go a long way towards redressing any historic criticisms. However, the findings of GP educators suggest that practical progress is slow and, despite the best intentions of the ruling bodies and much honest effort, dysfunctional SHO posts are still alive and well (Kelly and Murray, 1997).

An authoritative study of vocational training (Hayden, 1996) reflected the urgency of reviewing the relevance of the hospital-based period and the need to shift the emphasis in the direction of practice-based learning, with greater integration of the components of training. The way forward has been opened up. Local initiatives are piloting innovative hospital posts (Savage *et al.*, 1997) and a 50/50 division between hospital and practice (Savage *et al.*, 1996).

The most radical recommendation to date came from the ACO which in 1997 proposed a policy, in line with the WHO Charter for General Practice in Europe (WHO, 1995), that GP training should be substantially based in general practice for the full three years, with periods of hospital experience being commissioned on a basis of identified need (Orme-Smith, 1997).

This must give warning signals. If basic training for general practice is to be progressively withdrawn from the hospital setting and relocated to the practice or other community setting, e.g. public health medicine (JCPTGP, 1996), a SHO manpower crisis is brewing. For hospital trusts the best defence against this is to cherish their GP trainees.

As far back as 1990 a visionary GP leader proposed a list of criteria for developing a better quality experience for SHOs (Styles, 1990). These are widely accepted by consultant hospital teachers, but putting them into effect requires commitment and monitoring:

- the SHO's contract should specify the education content of a post and how it will be fulfilled
- each consultant's contract should quantify the teaching obligation
- protected time for learning should be identified
- teaching and assessment methods should be agreed between teacher and learner

- the specific core competences to be acquired in a given post should be agreed by the junior and the consultant, and attainment of these reviewed through regular discussion of progress.

Much has changed since these words were spoken and their realization is within our grasp.

Content	Domain
Teach good clinical material	Knowledge
Emphasize clinical skills, practical procedures, communication skills	Skills
Emphasize positive values/beliefs towards GPs	Attitude
Teach epidemiological perspective, reflecting on differences between hospital and community prevalence, possibilities of preventive approach and health promotion	Knowledge, skills and attitude
Demonstrate complementarity of hospital and primary care	Attitude
Indicate how you would like to see the GP use your facility	Behaviour
Summarize what you would like to see the best GP know about your specialty	Skills and knowledge
Reflect on why it is that your facility sometimes appears to be used inappropriately by GPs	Behaviour and attitude
Model communication skills when talking to relatives	Skills and attitude
Help SHO trainees identify their own educational needs and how to meet them	Knowledge and skills
Encourage SHOs to speculate on the GP perspective of a problem	Attitude
Encourage research and project work, literature and library use and publication	Skills
Model and discuss team work and management issues	Knowledge, skills and attitude

Figure 12.1 Suggestions to consultants for an educational programme for SHOs. Methods may include one or more of the following: didactic 'bedside' tutorial; case discussion, project, journal club, day-release; peer review, appraisal, evaluation, counselling; GP input to hospital teaching: encouragement and affirmation (showing the value of primary care as a specialization) and facilitating appropriate exposure to GP work.

Criteria	Methods
1 Quality of clinical teaching at the 'bedside', seminars etc	a Questionnaire: (i) structure, (ii) process
2 Extent to which learning time is protected (library/release/study leave)	b Data collection, timesheet, log diary
3 Relevance to general practice	c Dialogue one-to-one, or in a group, or peer review
4 Emphasis on communication skills with patient and team	d Video/audio recording
5 Involvement with GP during hospital post	e Assessment forms
6 Consultant attitudes to GP education	f Exam results
7 Workload	g Audit (project work, critical review)
8 Achievement of clinical competence	h Self-assessment; use of interactive computer or distance learning
9 Commitment to task	
10 Agreed educational objectives for the post	
11 Living conditions (amenities, accommodation, food)	

How to apply the above criteria:

Aspect assessed	Criteria	Method
SHO post	2, 3, 7, 10, 11	a(i), b, c
Consultant	1, 4, 6, 8, 9, 10	a(ii), c, d, e, g
SHO/trainee	4, 5, 8, 9, 10	a(i), a(ii), b, c, d, e, f, g, h
GP input	1, 3, 4, 5, 8, 9, 10	a(i), a(ii), b, c, d, e, g

Figure 12.2 Template for accrediting SHO posts.

Evaluation of the hospital training situation

A course organizer may be involved in the processes of accrediting, inspecting or evaluating SHO posts and will almost certainly have some part in selecting or assessing SHO trainees. Helpful advice on participating in hospital visits is offered by Hand (1994). The scheme in Figure 12.2 is offered as an aid to planning such activities – initially, opportunistically, or at regular intervals.

Exercise 17

1 In what ways does your region monitor the educational needs of SHO trainees?

2 At what points in vocational training does selection take place?

3 Who is responsible for selection for:
   (i)   entry into the scheme?
   (ii) hospital rotations/posts?
   (iii) training practice?

4 What criteria apply?

5 What is your role (in relation to SHO trainees) in:
   (i)   selection?
   (ii) monitoring/assessment?
   (iii) teaching?
   (iv) guidance and support?

Part 5

Managing vocational training

Overview

Even managers find it difficult to define the limits or summarize the core content of management. This should give us, as GP teachers, a degree of empathy with them. Increasingly we are 'buying-in' their expertise for the benefit of our practices, and some of it is rubbing off on us.

Course organizers have particular needs in this area. The small-scale, decentralized nature of the vocational training scheme, limited resourcing and the diversity of attendant activities (as illustrated by attempts to define our job description) result in the necessity to be our own managers.

The questionnaire on the early needs of course organizers provided evidence of our qualms about the task of managing the vocational training scheme in general and the day-release course in particular. Chapter 13 explores a variety of issues related to managing people, resources and change.

Less predictably, the survey showed that many course organizers wanted to know more about research so that they could advise trainees about their projects. For this reason, and because research issues impinge on audit, critical reading and library use, it is included here in Chapter 14, under the general theme of 'informatics', that is, managing information.

Practicalities such as financial arrangements, and inspection visits of various kinds, are further sources of anxiety. There is wide variation between regions, but some generalizations can be made. These form the basis of the chapter on the administrative tasks of the course organizer. Managers insist they can distinguish between management and administration, but some overlap is unavoidable. A database of selected information concludes Part 5.

Management is a derivative, interdisciplinary subject. Therefore much of this material will have as much (or as little) relevance to teachers and practitioners in all areas of health care as it has to the course organizer and the vocational training scheme.

Reading precepts about management will not make you proficient in it. We will not all become 'one-minute managers'. See how you get on with being a 'two-session manager' instead.

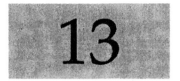

The two-session manager

Introduction

'You can run a consultation, you can run a practice, you can run a course.' (Anonymous course organizer)

Course organizers have a tendency to take on more and more tasks. Is this because they are good managers and can make room for them, or because they just can't say no? The high turnover among course organizers and the resulting problems of recruitment have not all been solved by improved conditions. A high proportion of course organizers admit to experiencing stress, with its damaging consequences on professional and family life. Course organizing is a time-consuming occupation which can easily become an obsession.

The questionnaire for new course organizers discussed in Chapter 1 highlighted management as an area in which they felt unprepared and under-resourced. Since all were experienced GPs and trainers, this implies a lack of management perspective among GPs in general – or could it be that it is mostly bad managers (who can't say no) who go into course organizing?

Many suspect that the mystique of management is maintained by management consultants for reasons of survival. As adult learners and educators, we all bring a wealth of experience and ability which is the foundation for skill building and growth. Managing is not about acquiring new knowledge, but about reflecting on what we do and how we can do it smarter, rather than harder.

Management considerations don't solve problems in course organizing. They help formulate the problems which arise, provide a framework of response and may contribute to avoiding some pitfalls. As with counselling, this cannot be learned from a book. This chapter summarizes the management aspects of course organizing. Although it is not a curriculum for teaching management to trainees it should help in constructing one.

Management principles relate to three main areas: people, resources and change.

People management

'Management is about people.' (Samuel, 1987)

Roles

The way people relate to their colleagues and perform their own role in an organization determines how effective they will be. These role relationships are chiefly affected by team work and leadership.

Team work happens when individuals work together to accomplish more than they would on their own (Woodcock, 1979).

'A team is an energetic group of people who are committed to achieving common objectives, who work well together and enjoy doing so and who produce high quality results.' (Francis and Young, 1979)

Factors influencing team work

According to McDerment (1988), the following have a good influence on team work:

- clear objectives – agreed goals
- openness and confrontation
- support and trust
- co-operation and conflict resolution
- sound procedures
- leadership
- regular review
- individual development
- sound intergroup relations.

Leadership is the ability to influence the thinking, the attitudes and the behaviour of co-workers or subordinates in some desired direction (Ends and Page, 1977).

Functions of leadership

These include:

- establishing, communicating and clarifying goals
- defining and negotiating roles
- planning activities

- setting standards of performance
- giving feedback to individuals and groups
- coaching and supervising
- initiating and enthusing
- being a role model
- influencing the climate of the group.

Leadership is characterized by:

- willingness to invest time and to provide continuity from day to day
- having strong feelings concerning attainment of goals
- an ability to focus on essentials.

As a course organizer your role of leadership in team work is exercised in:

- the day-release course with the trainees
- the trainers' workshop with the trainers (although frequently you are more of an *ex officio* member or resource person)
- the vocational training scheme with other course organizers.

Guidelines for team work and leadership

1 Be accessible – do not avoid your team.
2 Keep colleagues informed by giving clear and comprehensible instructions.
3 Provide opportunities to participate in decisions affecting them.
4 Allow airing of grievances – do not suppress criticism.
5 Give feedback about work achieved.
6 Encourage innovation and feedback.
7 Leadership and team work go hand-in-hand. The team may rotate the leadership role. Leaderless teams frequently malfunction.

Leadership and team work concepts and skills should be communicated specifically to the trainees, since their future roles will entail both. The Belbin Self-Perception Inventory is a useful tool for exploring an individual's team role or style when functioning in a team (Belbin, 1991).

Multiprofessionalism: an approach to working and learning

One neglected area of teamwork in medicine is interdisciplinary working and learning. Everyone asserts that it is a good thing but no-one seems to be very clear about what to do about it. It has been the subject of various substantial reports (for example Jones, 1996, SCOPME, 1997) and it received the endorsement of the GMC (1995). It appears to be at an early stage in development.

Early experiments in Exeter (Jones, 1996) documented the difficulties in implementing effective programmes – those of setting common goals, protected time, coordination and parity of representation between the respective professions. An attempt at joint training days involving social work students in Northern Ireland, based on discussing case histories, met with limited success. Selection of suitable cases was difficult and much time was spent getting the two groups to listen to one another rather than to focus on perceptions of the other based on stereotypes. It appeared that every social work student had at some time suffered at the hands of a doctor whilst none of the GP trainees had had the experience of a personal social worker. The resultant discussions were considered useful. Introducing other groups to this exercise was considered to be too daunting to attempt in the time available. A simpler approach was to invite tutors from related disciplines to resource sessions for registrars on the role and function of the respective members of the primary care team. The General Medical Council recommends that the multidisciplinary process should begin at undergraduate level. This will be facilitated by the trend for medical schools to become part of broadly based faculties of health science as in Southampton and Dundee.

Meanwhile, the subject is littered with terminology and nuance, fine distinctions being drawn between such concepts as multiprofessionalism; multidisciplinary, interdisciplinary and joint working; learning, education and training. A special interest organization has been formed – the Centre for the Advancement of Inter-Professional Education (CAIPE). In its evidence to the SCOPME working party it stated that 'interprofessional education is about people learning with, from and about one another'.

For the time being it is clear that health care is increasingly provided by multidisciplinary teams. Doctors are expected to work constructively within such teams and to respect the skills and contributions of colleagues (GMC, 1995). This is clearly a curriculum issue for vocational training. It is probable, however, that the greatest advances will be made at the level of continuing professional development as a result of reforms in regulations governing continuing education for GPs and incentives towards practice-based CME.

Communication skills

This complex area of interpersonal skills is fundamental to all our concerns as doctors, whether we are dealing with our learners, peers or patients, and in whatever capacity – teacher, manager or clinician. The skills are highly transferable. If we master them and communicate them to our learners much will have been achieved. Three deserve to be highlighted – assertiveness, mediation and persuasion.

ASSERTIVENESS

Assertiveness is nothing to do with authoritarianism or being a bully. It is a cluster of skills which is vital in professional and personal life, and is rooted in justice and clear communication. It includes:

- maintaining and protecting personal rights
- recognizing the rights of others
- making reasonable requests
- withstanding unreasonable requests from others
- handling unreasonable refusals
- avoiding unnecessary conflict
- communicating your own position confidently and openly.

Assertiveness is an important ability which trainees can be helped to practise.

MEDIATION

Mediation draws on the skills of counselling, facilitation, assertiveness and leadership in a conflict between two parties or within a group. It begins with recognizing that conflict is a natural part of significant relationships. Properly managed it offers opportunities for creative change. It should be invoked early in a dispute since mediation at the stage of terminal breakdown of a relationship is futile. It should address any disparity of power between the parties, facilitate each to confront the other with the problem as perceived, analyse the issues and work on them in a step-by-step process of problem solving to establish areas of agreement. Mediation may end with the drawing up of a contract.

The need for this can arise for the course organizer when an SHO trainee has a problem with the hospital hierarchy, or a practice trainee has a problem with the trainer. As course organizer you are well placed to mediate in both situations by virtue of your non-statutory, loosely defined but broadly based role in vocational training. You should be careful to maintain:

- independence from the parties to the conflict (not necessarily neutrality)
- credibility
- a grasp of the issues
- awareness of the process issues, e.g. the power balance or a hidden agenda
- commitment to identifying and solving problems through listening, dialogue and consensus.

PERSUASION

Persuasion is a communication skill based on proper authority in relation to other people by virtue of contract, specialist knowledge or awareness of valid goals, e.g. to persuade the trainees to undertake an unaccustomed task. It can be compared with the GP's role in the consultation and involves the:

- identification of issues through listening and dialogue
- exploration of the other's point of view
- discussion of agreed options and consequences
- information input
- formulation of an agreed plan.

Much useful information on communication skills may be found in *The inner apprentice* (Neighbour, 1996), *The doctors' communication handbook* (Tate, 1997) and a brief book of cartoons and wisdom, *Communicating with the public* (Kindred and Goldsmith, 1997).

Interviewing and selecting

Course organizers do a lot of this, mostly as part of a panel:

- selecting trainees for the scheme
- helping trainers to select a trainee
- participating in selection panels for hospital posts
- taking part in special situations especially at regional level, e.g. appointing of trainers, audit co-ordinators and new course organizers.

Shortlisting is an important preliminary. Usually there is a legal requirement to agree and write down the criteria for shortlisting in advance, e.g. minimum qualifications for the post. Discrimination on the grounds of race, gender or religion must be excluded. Shortlisting is frequently delegated to an administrator. This is a mistake. It determines the ground rules of subsequent interviews. As a key participant you should seek to influence decisions about shortlisting criteria.

The interview

Interviewing panels are frequently large and intimidating. Being courteous, addressing the candidate by name and not being too solemn (without being flippant) go a long way to getting the best out of the interviewee.

In GP-related hospital posts you may be asked to take the chair as the GP representative. You may find that you can be more influential if you do not take this role. The chair should be impartial. If you are chairman you can always ask a supplementary question, but not necessarily be able to ask questions in rotation with the others on the panel. Make sure that the ground rules are agreed with the panel beforehand, together with details about timing, scoring, how rigorous to be and whether to allow discussion between interviews.

It is customary to conclude by asking the candidate if he or she has any questions for the panel. Discussion of all candidates may follow but it is customary to ask each interviewer to draw up a league table or score card prior to this discussion.

The conclusion is usually a fairly arithmetic exercise. Unanimity is best, followed by voting and then tie-breaks in which another vote follows a debate.

Do not be afraid to leave posts vacant and re-advertise if no candidate seems to be up to your standard. Remember to keep your notes, because there may be appeals.

Guidelines for interviewing

Be wary of cracking jokes and never humiliate the candidate. Asides are distracting and unfair. You are not there to impress the others or the candidate and questions should be concise and prepared. Do not hesitate to re-phrase the question if the candidate has not understood it.

In questioning, retain control. Interrupt if the candidate embarks on a monologue. It is not an oral exam: you are not evaluating a subject but a person. If candidates are numerous, try to keep to some standardized questions.

Interviewing is an exercise in (true) assertiveness, involving a clear, unemotive dialogue with a respect for dignity and justice.

Be familiar with the job description, and be sure of what *you* want to know about *this* candidate. Read the CV for evidence of values and attitudes, but beware of references because they cannot be standardized. Some panels only allow references to be seen after all candidates have been interviewed and rank ordered.

Keep notes on all candidates' performance – how and why they impressed or disappointed you – with some form of numerical scoring to enable you to make your final ranking. Be particularly attentive to fairness with the first and last 20% of candidates, and make sure that your goal posts do not shift.

Appraisal of trainees

In the management setting appraisal is the periodic joint assessment, by the manager with one of his team, of the strengths and weaknesses of that team member's contribution towards attaining team objectives and the factors influencing it. This definition precludes a one-sided, judgemental approach and examines the setting as well as the person. For course organizers this usually applies to interviewing the trainee at intervals throughout the period of training.

A proper appraisal has the following characteristics:

- it is related to formative assessment in reviewing the trainee's progress
- it contributes towards evaluation of the course, i.e. the course organizer's self-assessment as an educator

- it may encompass educational audit and counselling
- it examines the educational opportunities and how they are being used
- it generates a record of objectives set and met
- it is particularly useful with regard to SHO trainees who are undertaking a succession of posts, because it provides continuity and a cumulative record of experience
- it provides opportunities for personal and other problems to be raised and responses to be planned, agreed and reviewed.

While it depends on the enthusiastic implementation by one person as co-ordinator, it is fostered by the co-operation or participation of others involved in the trainee's progress (SCOPME, 1991).

Guidelines for trainee appraisal interviews

... a process that is confidential (except in defined circumstances), primarily educational and developmental, and designed to help the individual to progress.' (Oxley, 1997)

1 Start early in the training period to establish the aims of appraisal.
2 Appraisal is a continuing, periodic process.
3 There should be a statement of aims and how to measure them.
4 There should be a cumulative structured record of appraisal.
5 The trainee should be involved in setting goals and reviewing his progress.
6 The course organizer should give feedback (remember 'Pendleton's Rules').
7 The course organizer may invite feedback about the course (try to avoid being defensive).
8 The trainee should be helped to express any problem he or she has.
9 Open questions help – this is a consultation.
10 Watch for signs of stress.
11 Make a contract about confidentiality, trainee access to the appraisal record and who should hold the record.
12 The course organizer should not seek to be the trainee's personal counsellor.
13 Appraisal takes time.

Liaison

Although as course organizer you may operate in a relatively autonomous fashion, even within a small team setting, your role as educational overseer suggests that it is important to maintain good lines of communication with all the other individuals and groups who are involved in the vocational training scheme: the trainers (especially the trainers' workshop), the hospitals and consultants who teach trainees, the regional director and associates at 'head office' and the course secretary. It is generally agreed that the course organizer should co-ordinate the different elements of vocational training at local level (Hayden, 1996).

Liaising with the trainers' workshop

A good relationship with the trainers is particularly important. You need to clarify your own relationship with this group in order to function effectively in it. Variation in the course organizer's involvement is wide. There may be more than one workshop relating to the day-release course, especially in urban catchment areas. Some course organizers are *ex officio* members, entitled to be present but little else. Sometimes he may be the *de facto* convenor. There is much to be said for a separation of function, with the course organizer relating closely with the convenor and attending as a resource person.

The aims of the trainers' workshop include:

- being a forum for trainers to meet for mutual help and support
- educating trainers and especially building skills and resources
- planning the group's training activities for the year
- developing a co-ordinated approach to vocational training by trainers and the course organizer in areas such as curriculum, projects and trainee exchanges
- developing programmes of trainee assessment
- exploring problems arising in training.

Cultivate your relationship with the trainers' workshop: it is among your chief resources, but don't try to run it if you have any alternative.

For the trainers, benefits of such a liaison include:

- the input of an independent, honest broker
- gaining a resource person with educational overview, group-work and process skills
- a complementary view of the trainees' progress and co-ordination of assessment methods
- the opportunity to compare notes (with a caveat about confidentiality)
- avoidance of duplication of effort
- the possibility of division of labour, e.g. identifying subject areas appropriate to the day-release course
- possibilities for involvement with the day-release course.

For the course organizer, the benefits include opportunities to:

- build up a good relationship with the training practices and to air problems
- recruit individuals to resource day-release course sessions
- build up a resource body for day-release course activities, e.g. mock exam, OSCE
- gain new ideas for programmes

- sort out trainee problems
- identify trainees' needs, e.g. practice swop, integrate modules and co-ordinate practice work with group work
- counteract personal feelings of isolation
- identify future course organizers.

Liaising with consultants and training hospitals

Ideally the course organizer relates to one local general hospital with enlightened, educationally oriented consultants. Many course organizers have to relate to widely dispersed hospitals of various sizes, and a body of consultants who feel harassed and are otherwise preoccupied.

To create a situation where SHO trainees receive both an educational experience of worth and also possible release from ward duties to attend the day-release course, you need to have the hospital and its staff on your side. This is frequently a problem (*see* Part 4).

Liaising with the regional directors

Among other things, the course organizer is the regional director's local representative. Many course organizers function in relative isolation, far from head office.

A few years ago, during a particularly bleak summer holiday, I visited a friend who is a sales representative in the west of Ireland, to pass a rainy afternoon. 'How do you manage here?' I asked. 'The roads are terrible, it rains all the time and the phone system is antiquated.' 'I do okay!' he replied. 'The roads keep the traffic down, the rain keeps the tourists away, and the phone system keeps head office out of my hair.'

An effort must be made to keep good lines of communication with head office. They employ you and they have resources you need. Many aspects of the day-release course require regional effort, e.g. core days and residential modules. The regional director's concerns are different from yours, being related to such things as policy, planning, budgeting, CME, standards, inspections, the JCPTGP and accountability to the Postgraduate Council.

If you are in Scotland you will already be (associate) regional director. Mostly the director is happy to see the course organizer getting on with the job, producing a rational and balanced programme, and keeping him informed. A brief written annual report of your course is generally appreciated. You can be a resource to him in consultation, planning, inspection of practices or hospital posts and selection procedures.

Liaising with the course secretary

The course secretary is invaluable, unless you can type and use a word processor, have your own personal photocopier and vast supplies of copy paper, a prodigious memory and lots of spare time. She hears more about the trainees than you do; she may know where they are hurting (and, indeed, where they are) when you don't. If you are the guide on the vocational training package tour, she is the travel agent. Her area of responsibility can be expanded to assisting with programme preparation, locating, briefing and ensuring payment of resource people and marshalling your other resource needs.

The provision of course secretaries is variable. Some course organizers have none. Others could go fishing and leave everything to her. Almost invariably she has other duties, so be aware of the balance of demands on her time and patience. Be realistic about deadlines – things take time. A secretary whose time is always respected will perform miracles in an emergency.

Survival pack

Unlike other activities in people management, the management of stress is usually an individual activity. The manager sorts out his own business, and may also be an initiator or resource person for his team in this area. There is a growing awareness of the value of self-help groups for people who work in situations of isolation and stress. The following guidelines come from the 10 most common responses by US managers in order of frequency (Burke, 1971).

1 Change lifestyle habits to build stress resistance.
2 Compartmentalize home and work life.
3 Take regular physical exercise.
4 Talk it through on the job with peers.
5 Withdraw physically from the situation.
6 Change to engrossing non-work activity.
7 Talk it through with spouse.
8 Review workload.
9 Analyse the situation and alter strategy.
10 Change to different work task.

Sources of stress reported by Shapiro and Clawson (1982) were given the acronym 'PACEING':

P – physical – noise, posture, clothing, fatigue
A – affective – anger, depression, anxiety, conflict
C – cognitive – overload, conflict, decision making
E – environmental – heat, ventilation, colour

I – interpersonal – colleagues, clients, family
N – nutritional – caffeine, alcohol, snacking, smoking
G – genetic – type-A personality

Each identified stressor may be matched with a stress management technique to avoid *burnout*. This has been defined as, *'A syndrome of physical and emotional exhaustion involving the development of a negative self-concept, negative job attitudes and a loss of concern and feeling for clients'* (Pines and Maslach, 1978).

Resource management

Managing time properly is one of the best ways to reduce stress. If you feel you haven't time for important tasks, either you are too busy or the tasks are not important to you.

How you use your time is related to your personality, priorities, cognitive style and individual situations in your professional and personal life.

Having two jobs – general practice and course organizing – with open-ended, unrestricted job descriptions, is an explosive mixture. Time management prescriptions do not alter this. If you do all the things time managers advise you to do, you may end up working harder and feeling a failure. Scan the items of advice for the ones which are easy. Try them out, but remember that trying out new things takes time. Consider trying out a few of the more unlikely-looking ones in turn.

The Irish College of General Practitioners suggested some guidelines (ICGP, 1991):

- 'work smarter, not harder'
- develop a personal sense of time, perhaps by keeping a diary of time spent
- plan ahead: a day (on paper) – jobs that must be done today
  - jobs that should be done today
  - jobs that can wait
  - 'time for me'

  a week (in diary)
  a month (in diary/calendar)
- prioritize tasks: (a) urgent, important – do it now, giving as much time as necessary
  - (b) non-urgent, important – assign time later
  - (c) urgent, unimportant – do now quickly
  - (d) non-urgent, unimportant – ignore?
- make the most of your best time: use it for vital tasks, allow quiet time for thinking, planning and don't forget family, friends and hobbies
- capitalize on marginal time – read while you travel and allocate short tasks for short spaces
- avoid clutter
- do it now: set deadlines and finish what you start

- learn to say no: don't let others steal your time and avoid over-commitment
- use the phone – be brief, don't visit if you can write a postcard, and don't write if you can telephone. Fax is fast, inexpensive and you retain your document. E-mail is rapidly becoming an imperative, with the possibility of instant, inexpensive recorded dialogue and network communication. The virtual committee – one which never physically meets – is a virtual reality.
- delegate: give your secretary standard letter templates and the key to your filing cabinet. Don't reinvent the wheel. If someone else has done it before and it works, copy it
- meetings – cut them down, keep them short and use chairing skills
- welcome problems – they'll find you anyway
- anticipate and handle interruptions. Some things are beyond your control.

Meetings

These are not optional extras. They are part of modern working practice and essential to team work evaluation and planning.

Meetings over a meal are often an excuse for a meal. They are prolonged, untidy and full of interruptions. Have the meeting and have the meal later. If the meetings are full of social conversation, perhaps you should be having a team outing and a separate meeting. Meetings should be purposeful and businesslike. For the course organizer the main meetings are with fellow course organizers, the regional directors, the trainers' workshops, the trainees' representatives and hospital-based teachers.

Others will seek to draw the course organizer into committees for district functions because he is a GP whose name has become known to the hospital and community services – audit groups, postgraduate centre management group and so on. Do not let them take over your life.

Dunham (1988) suggested the following guidelines about meetings:

- keep them to the minimum
- calendar well in advance
- send minutes and agenda one week in advance
- keep the agenda short
- clarify the aims. Is the meeting to discuss points of view, review progress or make decisions?
- state who is responsible for each item at the end of the session
- act promptly on decisions
- keep to stated starting and ending times
- keep a file for each separate committee (well weeded to avoid clutter).

Marshalling resources (people, topics and materials)

Keep a brief record of all day-release course sessions. Each successful session is another resource next time round, while each 'unsuccessful' session needs a post-mortem: don't just bury it. Build up lists of resource people: GPs, consultants, non-medical experts, community leaders, the local institute of higher education (university, college of education, technical college etc.), chamber of commerce, community voluntary and self-help groups, even the patient or individual with a 'story to tell'. There are plenty of people with something of value to communicate to the GP trainee, and the course organizer will learn a thing or two in the process.

Watch out for 'new' topics – the MRCGP examiners do this too – by keeping an eye on the press, magazines, television and the editorials of the journals. These reflect current concerns in society and may find a place in your programme.

Among your resource people are the pharmaceutical representatives. Increasingly they have non-promotional wares to offer such as high-quality videos, workshops and literature. They have even been known to help with the 'works outing' (or 'stress management fieldwork' as it appears in some programmes).

Your basic office needs are a filing cabinet, book shelf, card index, a large waste bin and a writing space which is periodically cleared. The marshalling of materials can be a major problem for course organizers. Keep on top of things by scanning, abstracting (on 6 × 4 inch filing cards), filing, weeding and shredding. Many retiring course organizers find they have an extra living room when the bonfire goes out. The following guidelines for desk efficiency are taken from a very useful little book called *Get organised* (Pollar, 1993):

- throw out or recycle as much as possible
- decide immediately, don't shuffle papers
- place like things together
- label files and binders using broad, simple headings
- keep close to you only the things you use frequently
- complete items once you begin
- make follow-up notes in a diary, project or to-do list only
- refile and replace things quickly
- keep it simple
- clear your desk at the end of each day.

Practical arrangement for the day-release course

With your programme prepared and your resources marshalled, remember the important details:

- as Maslow said, higher order human activity (self-actualization, self-realization) demands lower order biological comforts (heat, light, air, breaks, space and coffee)

- make sure the space is booked
- review next week's arrangements (and the following week's) this week
- decide whether the trainees need preparatory work
- ask yourself whether the speaker needs further details
- prepare handouts, overhead transparencies and any special equipment
- preview the day's programme briefly the night before. Write 'the order of service' (including the announcements)
- review the day's programme briefly the night after, and write down any lessons learned
- file notes, handouts and materials for future reference.

Problem solving and decision making

Managers, like GPs, manage messes. Before we get round to problem solving and decision making, there is the intermediate stage of problem setting – *'the process by which we define the decision to be made, the ends to be achieved, the means which may be chosen'* (Schön, 1983).

Having untangled the cluster of problems, they may be tackled in a more or less logical way. This process resembles the GP consultation except that many people may be involved and the prescriptive remedy cannot simply be dispensed by someone else.

Decision making is not about decisiveness. It is a stage in the reflective process of problem solving. The individual's cognitive style will influence the methods and pace of the process. Relevant qualities on the part of the decision maker include:

- the ability to assemble information in an orderly way
- an understanding of probability
- a willingness to discuss problems with peers and others involved in or affected by the process (RCGP, 1988). There is no experimental evidence for an independent variable called 'problem-solving ability' (Norman and Schmidt, 1992).

Decision making and innovation

Innovation relates to defining the goals of change and creating the conditions for realizing desired outcomes. Much decision making in the management setting relates to innovation. In the decision-making process, three elements have to be taken into account (RCGP, 1989).

1 The innovation – what are its advantages? Who is backing it and why? How complex is it and how disruptive might the transition be? What risks are involved, and can they be reduced by a pilot study before the final decision?

Consider:	clarify problem; ultimate objective; constraints; information requirement
Consult:	maximize available information, staff meetings
Crunch:	gather options; take decisions; write implementation plan
Communicate:	briefing on effects – what, whom, why; back up with written confirmation and implementation steps
Check:	run spot checks to monitor, review and correct

Figure 13.1 Decision taking – key actions (after Sargent and Wilkinson, 1980).

2 The people involved – what are the characteristics (flexibility, level of skills and commitments) of the group most affected? What is their track record on implementing change? Find out who are the opinion-leaders in the group and get them involved.

3 The organization – how will the decision affect role relationships? What is the organization's track record on implementing change? What procedures have to be applied to get a decision? How is the rate or extent of change to be monitored and controlled?

To summarize:

- don't make mountains out of molehills, make molehills out of mountains (problem setting)
- divide and rule (problem situations, not people!)
- assemble information in an orderly way
- what is the desired outcome, and are there secondary targets if the primary one is missed?
- decisiveness springs from the balanced, well-informed manager's assessment of probability
- discuss problems and listen to points of view
- try a simulation or pilot study
- do not bury 'wrong' decisions, analyse them.

Stages in decision making/problem solving and corresponding responses are summarized in Figure 13.2.

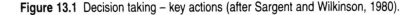

Management of change

One of the key differences between management and administration is in the area of change. Change is an essential feature of a vocational training scheme. The

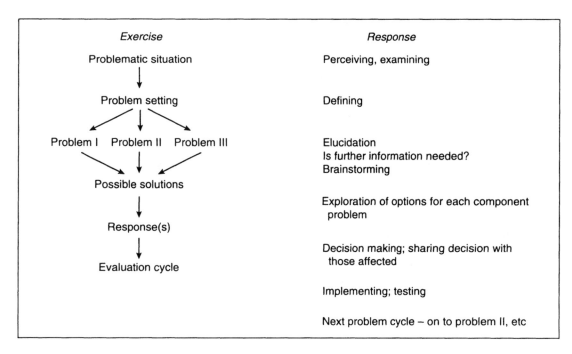

Figure 13.2 Summary of stages in problem solving and decision making.

immediacy of contact between course organizer and trainee means that the process of the day-release course is dynamic, trainee centred and responsive to new patterns of need. Educationally, the course organizer is a manager of change for, and within, the trainee group. Managerially, the course organizer is in a position to initiate change at district and regional levels in co-operation with the regional director. This may relate to regional policies, the hospitals and training practices and the trainers' groups.

The process of bringing about change is not simple. Exhortation and information are not effective agents of change, although they play a part.

Motivation

'We trained hard, but it seemed that every time we were beginning to form up into teams, we would be reorganized. I was to learn later in life that we tend to meet any new situation by reorganizing and a wonderful method it can be for creating the illusion of progress while producing confusion, inefficiency and demoralization.' (Caius Petronius, 66 AD)

Without motivation there is no real change and, as independent operators, course organizers have to be largely self-motivating. Occasionally directives from head office or a JCPTGP visit provide extra motivation. The other chief source of motivation is contact with other course organizers.

Cognitive dissonance – the realization that there is a gap between what we are doing and what we think we are doing – may prompt the cycle of change. If attitudes are negative towards a particular change, there may have to be coercion. However, change which results may quickly decay unless reinforced by practice, arising from improved performance, positive feedback and a feeling of gratification – the resolution of dissonance (Fox *et al.*, 1989).

If the changed state is maintained, the effort required diminishes and new patterns of behaviour are established. The change may then be subjected to the familiar cycle of evaluation and reformulation.

Failure to effect change arises from problems at any of these stages. It can be a demoralizing experience. Morale is a crucial factor, especially if there is partial or complete failure to achieve the goal of change. Good communication, clear definition of the goals and optimism are important if the participants are not to be immunized against future change. The stages of the cycle change and the corresponding activities or responses are summarized in Figure 13.3.

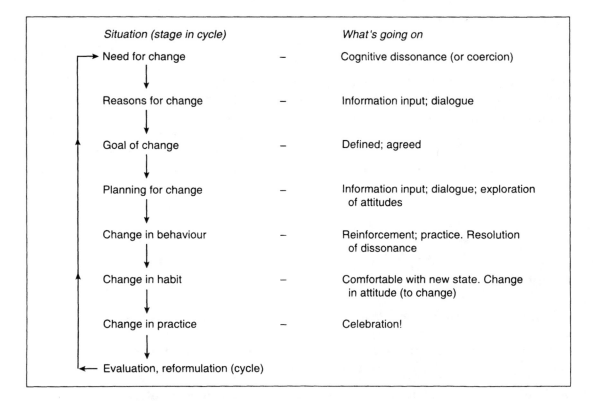

Figure 13.3 The cycle of change.

Guidelines for change

To bring about change, you will need to go through several stages: define the present state; describe the desired goal; analyse the difference (what steps need to be taken?); implement the transition; and finally consolidate the change. In implementation:

- ensure early involvement
- provide help in facing up to change
- avoid over-organizing
- communicate clearly and frequently
- focus on gaining commitment
- defuse perceived threats: see them as opportunities for dialogue.

Groups undergoing change are characterized by:

- high uncertainty, low stability
- stress
- energy
- control becoming a major issue
- looking to the past with longing
- conflict.

Audit and change

Irvine and Irvine (1997) described audit as: *'The process used by health professionals to assess, evaluate and improve the care of patients in a systematic way in order to enhance their health and quality of life.'*

This is an example of change within general practice in the UK which began as vision led and became crisis driven through contractual change. Unless people find it stimulating, rewarding and feasible, decay will set in. The audit cycle reflects the cycle of change. Essentially, audit generates information. This can be rewarding in itself, and is a productive feature of the vocational training scene. Information produced by audit provides the immediacy which helps education to flourish. Many curriculum themes for the day-release course are enhanced by the action-learning dimension of a preparatory audit-related activity. It demonstrates the cyclical pattern so pervasive in professional life (whether clinical, administrative or educational) and is essential to goal setting. Audit will be considered further in Chapter 14.

Exercise 18

1 What is *your* role in the trainers' workshop(s) you attend?

2 In what situations are your management skills tested?

Which skills need working on?

3 Think of a situation where you tried to effect a basic change in your practice or vocational training scheme. If it did not work, why not?

4 How do you incorporate management concepts in your curriculum for the trainees?

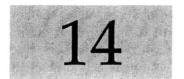

Informatics and information

Introduction

Informatics is the body of knowledge and practice related to the management of information. It does not have to be high-tech. At course organizer workshops I have, on occasions, raised the problem that I often feel that I am 'drowning in paper'. Accessing, storing and retrieving information is the key to our continuing education and professional development. It can help us to evaluate our work and lay the foundations for audit and research. As course organizers, we also have a responsibility to help trainees acquire the skills which will enable them to face the information explosion which will be an increasing feature of their professional life.

Research, literature and the library

Information processing

To help trainees to manage information, you may find it useful to explore for yourself the relevant tasks and skills. Becoming a course organizer is marked by a sudden increase in the amount of paper you have to deal with on all kinds of subjects: the trainers' workshop, regional issues (you are on the regional mailing list for everything, whether or not it directly affects you), postgraduate council proceedings, trainer selection committee proceedings, trainee selection, visitation matters of various kinds, hospital business such as vocational training rotations and SHO appointments, course organizer business (assessment material for SHO and practice trainees, day-release course materials and programmes), promotional material (from publishers, pharmaceutical companies and educational organizations, who all see you as the key to the trainee market), circulars and surveys (everybody wants to know your opinion on everything), your own CME stuff (as a GP and as a course organizer), and working documents (minutes, agendas, circulars, programmes, journals and resource materials).

Guidelines for handling paperwork

The following guidelines may be easier said than done:

- keep course organizing materials separate from personal and practice work documents
- delegate the organization of material
- deal with each document as it comes in
- abstract useful information on filing cards with standard headings, referencing source and location of original document
- have an active filing system – card index and cabinet files, clearly labelled and periodically reviewed and weeded
- use portfolios, diaries (preferably *one*), logs (again clearly labelled)
- have a phone extension on your desk
- keep personal computer/word-processor on a separate working surface – it takes up a lot of space and easily becomes inaccessible
- if you use a word-processor, organize and index the files/disks to allow easy access. Delete redundant material
- use open-side file boxes and keep journals off the floor and desk.

Pollar (1993) has produced a helpful book on the skills of managing papers, files and information.

The library – workshop or warehouse?

Information which is not accessible is not informative. If you want to hide information, put it in a library. Even the best library is only a warehouse unless you know how to unlock its access codes. The librarian is there to turn the warehouse into a workshop for your educational needs. Trainees who have not actively used the library by the end of vocational training are locked out for life. They should be encouraged to find out what resources are available so that they will know how to get the information they want. Make library use one of the educational objectives of the day-release course, by:

- direct teaching, with a session resourced by a librarian
- hands-on experience of literature search and database through use of manual, microfiche, computerized and on-line searches

- action learning through projects, audits and research to consolidate learning
- a demonstration of how to access library services remotely (how does the young principal in an isolated area obtain access to medical library services?)
- listing other kinds of database facilities available through RCGP, BMA, hospital pharmacy, accident and emergency (for toxicology)
- promoting awareness of economical use of library facilities, e.g. the cost of an on-line search.

Guidelines for literature search

Avoid the 'toilet-roll' approach to literature search which produces printout a mile long. Be specific about what you are looking for (subject, key words and synonyms and be aware of alternative spellings). Set limits to the search in the areas of language (e.g. English only), geography (e.g. UK only) and year (e.g. post-1995).

General resources include information bureaux (e.g. Age Concern), professional associations (e.g. Institute of Management) and libraries (public, university, post-graduate centre, RCGP, BMA, British Library etc.). You should be able to find most of what you want with proper use of library catalogues, bibliographies, abstracts and indexes, computer databases, official report literature (e.g. HMSO), circulars and statistical sources (e.g. from the Registrar General, with the caveat that statistics date quickly and are not comparable between countries). You may have problems, however, with foreign language or obscure publications (locating them via interlibrary loan or the British Library may take time) and theses (although the librarian should be able to help).

Specific library exercises and project work introduce the trainee to the library in a practical way. Figure 14.1 shows an example of such a learning task for trainees (from the Northern Ireland vocational training scheme).

Library – useful articles

Anderson UW (1988) How to set up a simple practice library. *Update*. **20**: 80–1.

Haynes RB *et al.* (1986) How to keep up with medical literature: VI. How to store and retrieve articles worth keeping. *Annals of Internal Medicine*. **103**: 978–84.

Henderson AS and Bosly-Craft R (1983) A simple system for references and reprints. *British Medical Journal*. **287**: 1448–9.

Mead M (1984) The trainees' library. *Trainee,* **March**.

RCGP (1988) *The practice library*. Royal College of General Practitioners, London.

Sellu DP (1986) A comprehensive bibliography database using a microcomputer. *British Medical Journal*. **292**: 1643–5.

MDEC Library: Self-assessment questions
General questions: F

Please answer these questions using the information given during your tour of the library or in the *Introduction to Stock and Services*. Return to the library issue desk when completed.

Practice scenario. A colleague has been conducting a smoking cessation clinic. One of the chronic smokers who attended has asked for information on a drug *Zyban* which was featured in a *Sunday Times* article on 7 September 1997. Being an American drug it does not appear in the *BNF* so she approaches you to find out more information [during your regular weekly visit to the medical library!]

1 Using the **INTERNET**.
   Click on the [Search] icon at the top of the screen. Click in the *Infoseek* search engine window. Type in: *ZYBAN* then click on Search.

   (a) How many Hits (relevant items) do you get? _____
   (b) Scroll down the screen and go into a newswire item site.
       Write down the generic chemical name of Zyban: _____
   (c) In a pharmacy website view and print out, if desired, a consumer guide to the use and side-effects of this drug.

2 Using the **MEDLINE** Database.
   Start the OVID software and load the MEDLINE database.
   When *Enter Subject* appears in the middle of the screen type in your subject heading. Complete 2 separate subject searches, taking all documents and all subheadings for each, on:

   BUPROPION
   SMOKING CESSATION

   (a) Then [Combine Sets]. How many references do you have? _____ .
       Use *View Set* to view the references, and select and print any of use.

3 Using the **COCHRANE LIBRARY.**
   Start the Cochrane Library CD-ROM software. Click on the search icon at the top left of the screen.
   Type in your subject heading:

   BUPROPION
   and start the search.

   How many references are retrieved in all of the Cochrane databases? _____

   View and print the reference to a 1996 article on the use of a sustained release preparation of this drug.

Figure 14.1 Learning task sheet: library use.

Information technology

'2000 generations ago humans began to use language
200 generations ago writing was invented
20 generations ago books were first printed
2 generations ago the computer was invented.' (Quoted in Collins, 1997)

Is it surprising, therefore, that so many of us are computer-shy (or phobic)? In 1996, a simple postal survey was carried out through regional representatives of the Association of Course Organizers. It indicated that:

- most course organizers make some use of computers, mostly simple word-processing for document preparation and the use of educative software
- some regions are introducing modem linkage between postgraduate centres and with the regional office
- very few regions provide significant training in information technology (IT) skills for course organizers
- there is very little IT training provided for trainees at the day-release courses: only 13 out of 44 courses provided more than two IT-related sessions for each intake of trainees.

Scottish regions appear to be most advanced in this field, with policies such as 'all training practices are computerized and trainees should routinely use the computer during consultations'.

There is some coherent curriculum development going on, and an increasing sense of urgency to establish IT firmly on the learning curriculum for all hospital and general practice trainees. This is essential preparation for current, not to mention future, working practice. IT applications relevant to general practice that are currently being developed and evaluated include telemedicine linkages and networks, distance learning and remote library access (Collins, 1997). The possibility already exists for 'virtual committees' which transact all their business by e-mail. It is possible to bring the practice clinical database to the GP at the bedside domiciliary visit.

Vocational training is about accelerated learning. For trainees at present the learning of IT skills appears to be under-developed. Clearly, there is much more to skilled use of IT than simply using the surgery computer for routine tasks. The range of topics might include:

- library facilities – print, microfiche, CD-ROM and on-line systems
- remote access to databases – on-line literature search, Internet and World Wide Web-site information
- manipulation of computer files – text, images, spreadsheets and e-mail
- use of commonly available hardware – copier-printer-scanner, fax and the potential use of smart card applications.

It is also important to be familiar with the ethical issues of security and confidentiality, and relevant legislation.

There are few areas of course organizing at present which cannot be adequately managed with manual systems, although this will undoubtedly change. If you regularly use a literature reference system with more than 200 file cards you would probably benefit from a computerized system.

In large schemes with a high turnover of trainees, a computer may be useful for storing and retrieving personal files, especially as formative assessment and appraisal become more sophisticated. This is governed by the provisions of the Data Protection Act (*see* Part 6). The computer is also becoming more popular as a teaching tool; the use of interactive disks in clinical and management problem simulations, for instance, tests knowledge and decision making on an individual or small-group basis. One example is PEP (Phased Evaluation Programme), which contains 60 MCQ and patient management problems on an interactive disk. The RCGP library has a catalogue of reference works available on CD-ROM. Every junior doctor and trainee should be encouraged to learn basic word-processing and computing skills.

Many training practices are well advanced in the application of computers to clinical care and practice management. They should be used as a resource for all trainees, and trainers with relevant expertise should be invited to the day-release course. Practice exchanges should be considered for those trainees in practices where computers are not routinely used; trainees in highly computerized practices would benefit from the exchange by seeing how practices manage without them!

Critical reading

'Critical reading is a process that has two major components – why and how.' (Macauley, 1994)

Critical reading is now a prominent feature of the MRCGP examination. This reflects a concern on the part of the examiners to be relevant and formative within a summative context. The intention is to build the habit of active reading, and the ability to form opinions which are based on fact and a critical evaluation of source material. It carries with it the dangers inherent in summative assessment, of putting people off for life, or making them confine their reading to scientific literature.

These tendencies can be corrected by keeping preparation for examinations in perspective, and incorporating an evidence-based approach to all course work.

The reading syndicate with group discussion – the journal club – has been a feature of hospital-based and vocational training for a long time. It needs to be actively managed, like any group task, with agreed rules on format and conduct.

Items to be reviewed and discussed should be purposefully selected and analysed in a structured fashion for content, method and message (*see* Figure 14.2). Creation of

Summary	Is it a concise statement of the topic(s) and conclusions?
Introduction	Does it provide a clear outline of the background to the topic?
Methods (design)	Is the sample size appropriate, and how was it selected?
	Is the study retrospective or prospective?
	What are its strengths, limitations and flaws?
Results	Is the presentation clear?
	Are the illustrations useful?
	Are the results significant, clinically and statistically?
Discussion	Is it relevant?
	Does it show what it claims, or are there false assumptions?
Further questions	Does it support other findings?
	Does it tally with my own experience?
	Does it have any implications for me?

Figure 14.2 Template for critical reading.

a variety of templates covering different approaches is itself a useful learning exercise which contributes to a grasp of evidence, issues and controversies, and leads to a sense of the development of thinking in specific areas.

A major problem area for journal clubs lies in the selection and organization of material. How do the members productively approach the task of assimilating the vast quantity of relevant publications? The technique for critical appraisal is fairly easily grasped, but trainees need tools to help them read selectively as well as critically and, at the same time, comprehensively. One such tool to govern the question of selectivity goes by the acronym 'READER' (Macauley, 1994):

Relevance (to general practice)
Education (will it change behaviour?)
Applicability (to practice)
Discrimination (is it valid, refereed; quality of source?)
Evaluation (worth presenting)
Reaction (file, mental note or forget it?)

Reasonable comprehensiveness may be achieved by applying the following guidelines:

* scan editorials in quality (refereed) journals related to general practice
* major review articles in quality journals on primary care themes
* reports of national and international collaborative trials
* data derived from classic prospective trials, e.g. Framingham Study
* research funded by high-profile bodies, e.g. Medical Research Council

- nationally agreed statements relevant to practice, e.g. British Thoracic Society asthma guidelines
- official reports on specific primary care themes, e.g. Forrest Report on screening for breast cancer
- public reports and government documents that influence health policy, e.g. white papers
- references that appear recurrently in a variety of reputable articles on a given topic
- health issues that have a high media profile.

Not all of these require critical appraisal in detail, but they provide landmarks to the territory in which trainees should have a grasp of evidence and be able to give informed opinions.

The reading trainee

Every region provides a book list of recommended texts for trainees. The course organizer and the trainers' workshop might help their trainees by making additions and deletions, and providing guidelines and indications of priority.

A simple reading list is a very blunt educational tool. It takes no account of the cognitive styles of the individual learners. Its value is enhanced by reading syndicates: the pooling of reading tasks and sharing of information within a group setting. Trainees frequently have to be reminded that there is very much more to the literature of primary care than the primary literature of research and learned journals.

Audit and research: the educational setting

In the UK it is now a requirement for trainers to ensure that their trainees experience audit in their practices, and it will soon be a contractual obligation on all GPs. The 'trainee project' is also a well-established feature of vocational training, and audit is on the training curriculum as a requirement for the summative assessment. It is specifically (although not exclusively) the responsibility of the trainer.

If we teach about audit and ignore research, we run the risk of devaluing audit and mythologizing research as something remote and apart from primary care. For prospective hospital specialists, there is provision of protected time, supervision and funding for research training. This has not been readily available to GP trainees, which in part accounts for the slow progress of general practice research and for the apparent reluctance of many GPs to embrace audit. Coining the phrase 'the Law of Inverse Opportunity', Denis Pereira Gray lamented the obstacles to carrying out GP-initiated research from within general practice (Pereira Gray, 1991). This is now being redressed with an increase in resources devoted to research training and primary care project funding. Even the prestigious Medical Research Council is embracing the need to sponsor research in, and on, primary care (MRC, 1997). '... *the MRC considers a detailed understanding of the methods of putting basic science into clinical practice to be at least as important as pushing back the frontiers of basic research*' (Radda, 1998).

The emphasis on audit and critical reading in the examination systems is intended to make clinical general practice increasingly evidence based and reflective. Unless audit and research are dealt with as educational issues there is a risk that the evidence-based element will predominate over the reflective.

Coles (1990) suggested that the accepted audit cycle might be educationally barren: '*It does not by itself provide the necessary conditions for people to learn through it. As it stands the audit cycle is a bureaucratic view of changing professional practice, not an educational one. It is concerned more with the control of people's actions than with helping them.*'

He quoted McWhinney's (1989) observation that medical people are only likely to change 'through a process of reflection, personal development and growth of self-knowledge' and the audit should be creating the conditions for this to happen. As a remedy he proposed that the audit cycle should be combined with a learning cycle (*see* Figure 14.3) so that the process does not begin with a set of received standards but with reflection on practice from which autonomously determined standards will emerge. Thus the workers own the process themselves, and there is no reason to believe that this should correlate with lower standards. He described a method of implementing this in the group setting, as used in the Wessex vocational training scheme, noting that such a peer review group should be led by someone with group process skills (Coles, 1990).

The advantage of this approach is that it shifts the focus from information gathering and systems change (the mechanistic view of audit) towards reflection on the assumptions which underlie general practice (the humanistic view). This reflects two competing or complementary views of research.

The first – *the empirical model* – is derived from the physical sciences (with their emphasis on observation and testing the hypothesis objectively and rigorously). General practice is a professional discipline rather than an applied science. It is therefore at two removes from the methodology of research which historically has served the pure sciences so well. It is based on the collaborative attempt by doctor and patient to resolve the practical human problems of the individual interacting in a complex way with the social setting. This requires a generalist, interdisciplinary approach. The empirical model of research lacks congruity with this setting. For practitioners, rigour is no substitute for relevance. This perceived lack of relevance, along with the historical lack of training, opportunity and resourcing for research in general practice, contributes to the dichotomy between audit and research. Good GPs might do audit, but they are unlikely to do research.

The second model is *qualitative research*. One interesting variant has been termed 'new paradigm research' or collaborative inquiry (Rowan and Reason, 1981). It may

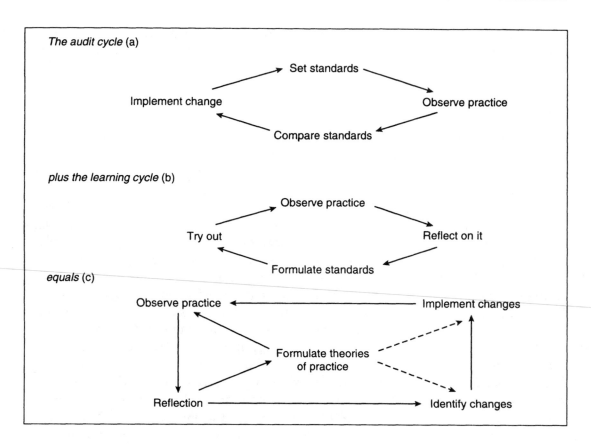

Figure 14.3 Fusion of the audit and learning cycles.

be seen as the third point of a triangle of autonomous enquiry which also comprises audit and empirical research. It is concerned with the investigation of dynamic human systems rather than static physical phenomena. If a statistical system is invoked it is more likely to be Beyesian than parametric. Groups of practitioners reflect on their own and each other's professional experiences and problems as adult learners. This 'reflection in action' creates a process whereby outcomes are discovered and tested as they arise. Learners experience and describe change as the process continues, and hypotheses can be postulated retrospectively. Insofar as there are 'investigators' and 'subjects', they both grow and change in their perspectives as they go along. This is reminiscent of the Balint group method. It incorporates elements of discovery, out-come results, peer review and affective learning through group interaction. This model challenges the empirical model – its emphasis on rigour, method, statistical validation of outcome, and its claim to be the exclusive research paradigm. As general practice educators, our reorientation from empirical to new paradigm research may be analogous to our transition from teacher-centred to learner-centred education.

Trainees' learning experiences in the area of research hinge on a few fundamentals:

- an ethos which includes research as a general practice activity. Few are currently encouraged to do research, and even fewer do it
- the demythologizing of research – it is not the monopoly of the ivory tower establishments or international journals; it is the process of finding rational answers to one's own questions, however small and simple
- morale – few people single-handedly achieve early success with easy publication of their first attempts. The disappointments of early experience are easily interpreted as failure, and a sympathetic mentor is vital
- statistics – few clinical researchers are statistical experts. Unfortunately many statisticians are based in teaching hospitals and seem remote. They are best approached once a protocol is formulated and before any clinical investigation has begun. Not all research requires statistical treatment. Audit, action research and collaborative enquiry models generally require little statistical back-up.

Every jobbing course organizer must be able to help trainees with audit and projects. Course organizers for whom research is not a personal priority can nevertheless discharge their function in relation to trainees by identifying an appropriate resource person, e.g. a partner in a designated research practice, who is willing to be available to help trainees.

Advice and training in research methods are available through university departments of general practice. These departments also have research fellowships or junior lectureships designed to get young doctors started. The RCGP Clinical and Research Division provides advice and some supportive services, including the funding of fellowships. Distance learning packages, many leading to postgraduate degrees, are now numerous. Established course organizers can now learn new skills more easily than in the past.

Research and development *'must stop being the eccentric pursuit of a few committed enthusiasts and start being an integral part of everyday professional practice'* (Mant, 1998).

The trainee project

This has been a widespread feature of vocational training for many years. One contributory factor was the establishment of the Syntex Award Scheme which operated for many years. Many faculties of the RCGP also have an award scheme, and the College has published a selection of award-wining trainee projects (RCGP, 1988).

There is now an expectation that the course will encourage and promote project work. Trainees should be encouraged to consider project work during the hospital phase of training. Information can be obtained from the regional director about funding for projects which have extraordinary resource requirements. Most projects are

Presentation	Is the format properly structured?
	Are aims, methods, results and illustrations presented clearly?
	Is the discussion of findings clear and adequate?
	Is there an adequate reference list (where appropriate) or bibliography?
Methodology	Are the aims clear and attainable?
	Is a pilot study required?
	Were controls necessary?
	Is there evidence of bias?
	Did statistical methods justify the conclusions?
	Were there ethical considerations?
Amount of work	What is a reasonable amount of work to be expected from a motivated trainee?
	Was it cost-effective?
Relationship to other work on same topic	Is there evidence of background reading?
	Has a literature survey been carried out?
	Have references been used effectively?
Relevance to GP	Is the project likely to have an impact on the attitudes of the trainee or his practice?
	Did the trainee, as a GP, appear to gain anything from carrying out the project?

Figure 14.4 Guidelines for formative and summative assessment of trainees' project (after Moran, 1990).

carried out within the resources of the teaching practice and under the supervision of the trainer.

With the increasing emphasis on assessment, it is important for the course organizer to be able to evaluate projects. There is so much common ground between instruction and assessment that a template for the latter may serve as a useful tool when briefing trainees or helping them with difficulties (*see* Figure 14.4).

What the course organizer can do: guidelines

The course organizer may promote the effective management of information by:

- including action learning and audit as regular features of the day-release course
- including a major project as a course objective
- helping trainees to think small and simple in project work
- encouraging literature-based and evidence-based approaches to clinical and managerial questions

- raising the profile of critical thinking and reading in the course
- identifying resource persons/bodies available (GP audit facilitators and those with a research interest to act as mentors, and regional resources such as university departments of general practice, medical librarians and statisticians)
- promoting the value of medical writing (putting pen to paper or fingers to keyboard initiates the flow of ideas and brings within reach the pleasures of publication)
- laying the foundations of methodology, by making sure that trainees know about critical reading, the audit cycle, library skills, word-processing and using a personal computer
- adopting the adult educator's perspective: seeing every crisis as a learning (research) opportunity, realizing that every individual has his own cognitive style, and encouraging everyone to identify his own questions and means of investigation.

15

Administration of
vocational training

Introduction

The effective delivery of any service relies on an efficient logistic base. This chapter deals with some practical matters relating to the organization of vocational training.

Although many course organizers have a high degree of autonomy and achieve competence in a wide range of activities within the vocational training scheme, none of us is self-sufficient. It is possible to function as a course organizer while having only a vague understanding of the funding arrangements and how regional and national structures interact. The extent to which course organizers are actively involved in the administration of resources varies widely between, and even within, regions. The same applies to involvement in the selection, inspection and approval of training posts in hospitals and training practices. Years may pass before a course organizer is personally confronted with a visitation by the JCPTGP, since such visitations, although regular, focus on sub-units of each region in turn. All these matters, however, will have to be faced sooner or later. The survey of needs (*see* Part 1) revealed that many course organizers felt they were poorly briefed about these issues.

How these matters are administered relates to the overall structure of each region. This chapter therefore begins with an outline of a 'generic' region, and ends with an account (contributed by Dr Paul Sackin, former secretary of the ACO) of the development of our chief resource body, the Association of Course Organizers. Among other things it represents our interests and contribution at national level.

The regional structure of vocational training

Reorganization in 1996 amalgamated the regional health authorities into a small number of regional offices of the National Health Service. For the purposes of administration of postgraduate education, however, the former regions continue to exist as 'deaneries'. Each has essentially preserved its own structure of dean of postgraduate medicine and regional committee for postgraduate medical and dental education. Its director and associate directors of postgraduate general practice education are the former regional/associate advisers renamed. It is impossible to provide a definitive and concise guide which applies to all regions, because of:

- variations in the size of regions
- different jurisdictions in England and Wales, Scotland, Northern Ireland and the Republic of Ireland
- the presence of more than one university medical faculty in some regions and thus perhaps more than one postgraduate dean and department of general practice
- variations in the size, distribution and location of the teaching unit, the day-release course. Most are in district postgraduate centres but some are in university facilities. In a few regions, such as Wessex, the sub-unit (or district) administrative functions have been devolved or contracted out to universities. They operate from a local campus of whatever university is best placed, or disposed, to offer suitable facilities.

An outline of the generic structure of vocational training in a mythical region in Great Britain is shown in Figure 15.1. It might have:

- a population of approximately 4 million
- 150 training practices and 200 trainers
- 150 registrars in the general practice year
- 250 hospital trainees identified for training: some on rotational packages, a smaller number on self-constructed schemes
- 12 day-release courses run by 30 course organizers.

The postgraduate dean is usually appointed by the university in conjunction with the health authority. He is the head of the (regional) council for postgraduate medical and dental education. The secretary of council is its executive officer. The council devolves much of its function to specialty subcommittees, the largest of which is the general practice committee. This represents the educational interests of all GPs and consists of GPs nominated by bodies such as the health authority or their component districts, the RCGP faculty board, the university department of general practice, the BMA/GMSC and the trainees' committee.

The Director of Postgraduate General Practice Education (the 'regional adviser') is the executive officer of the general practice committee. He is a principal in general

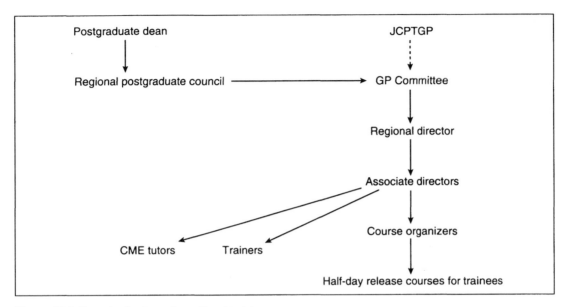

Figure 15.1 Generic structure of vocational training.

practice with a large sessional commitment (usually six sessions per week, but with increasing workload there is a move in the direction of full-time).

There is a supporting team of deputy directors (the 'associate advisers'). Each is a principal, with two or three sessions a week devoted to advisory functions, and with special responsibility for overseeing a 'portfolio' such as continuing medical education and GP tutors; vocational training and course organizers; assessment; IT development or planning. In some places non-medical experts, such as educationalists, are being appointed to advisory posts. This indicates that functions within the regional educational structure will not forever operate a general practitioner 'closed shop'.

Course organizers are GP principals with a contract of (normally) two sessions per week. They work alone, or in a small team of two to four, resourcing the educational and administrative aspects of vocational training in the district. In some larger centres the team leader may be an associate director or a course organizer whose duties are mostly in administration or co-ordination (scheme organizer). There may be a division of labour among course organizers: for example, one may be responsible for the day-release course, another for hospital liaison (the education and welfare of SHO trainees), while others may specialize in visiting and overseeing the training practices. There is a growing feeling that there should be a generic career path for GP teachers (Calman, 1995) based on the university model and perhaps requiring higher degree attainment for substantive posts such as director, course organizer and postgraduate tutor. There is a substantial body of opinion that GP teachers of all types have so much in common that their roles should be amalgamated to encompass undergraduate teaching, vocational training and continuing education.

Alternatively the roles of scheme organizer, course organizer and CME tutor may be combined under a generic title, such as 'district education adviser' (Orme-Smith, 1993).

In Scotland the functions of CME tutor and course organizer are already combined with those of the associate director. All course organizers are therefore associate directors but they carry out additional regional duties.

In the Republic of Ireland each scheme is totally autonomous. All are funded by the local health board, with or without additional assistance from a university. Each scheme has a steering committee representing trainers, trainees, hospital teachers, the health board (and university), the local faculty of the Irish College and the course organizer. Co-ordination at national level is through the Vocational Training Committee of the Irish College of General Practitioners. In the Republic of Ireland, course organizers enjoy the title of programme director. They conduct integrated three-year schemes (except in Sligo, where a four-year scheme incorporates one year in community health). The membership examination of the Irish College (MICGP) is the required certification for entry to practice.

In the UK each regional director is responsible, with the GP committee, for formulating and implementing provision of vocational training in hospitals and training practices, for supervising hospital training posts (a function of the Joint Committee delegated to the region), for appointing course organizers, trainers and approving training practices. He is responsible, therefore, for setting and maintaining the standards of vocational training. The region is accountable to the JCPTGP which has the duty to visit regions on a regular basis to inspect and make recommendations about standards and the implementation of training regulations and to accredit hospital posts. It can enforce compliance, the ultimate sanction being the withdrawal of recognition for training.

Other national institutions of relevance to vocational training are:

- SCOPME (the Standing Committee on Postgraduate Medical Education)
- COPMED (the Committee of Postgraduate Medical Deans)
- the Conference of Regional Advisers for the UK
- COGPED (the Conference of General Practice Educational Directors)
- SCPMDE (the Scottish Council for Postgraduate Medical and Dental Education, which co-ordinates the work of the five Scottish regional councils)
- WCPMDE (the equivalent body for Wales)
- the Northern Ireland Council for Postgraduate Medical and Dental Education (the equivalent body in Northern Ireland. It incorporates both regional and national characteristics)
- COAGP (the Conference of Academic Organizations in General Practice): an umbrella body which considers matters of public policy and developments of relevance to the various specialized interest groups in academic general practice – at undergraduate, vocational training, CME and research levels.

Exercise 19

Using the template provided in Figure 15.2, construct a profile of your region
The persons to whom you are accountable are:
Regional director ...
Associate director ...
Other ...

Outline Structure of Region _____

(Name)

Postgraduate dean   Name:

Postgraduate council   Chairman:

GP sub-committee   Chairman:

Regional director   Name:

Associate directors   Names:

Responsibilities
(e.g. vocational training, CME)...

Course organizers   Number of course organizers...

00   00   00   00   Number of venues/day-release courses...
How are course organizers deployed?...

Trainees   Number of trainees per course
in hospital...
in practices...
Number of trainers/training practices...
Total number of trainees...
Special regional features,
e.g. participation of medical school...
Approximate population of region...
Approximate number of GPs in region...

Figure 15.2 Outline structure of the region.

The fiscal structure of vocational training

Many course organizers have no worries about their budget. Their course secretary notifies details, such as fees for guest speakers at the day-release course, to the finance officer of the postgraduate council, who signs the cheques. Most, however, have to work with a more diverse structure. Questions inevitably arise concerning the funding of:

- special events, e.g. residentials and modules
- reimbursement of travel and subsistence expenses of trainees
- capital expenses, e.g. equipment
- salary and terms of service, e.g. the course secretary or scheme administrator
- petty cash for coffee etc.

Reforms in the early 1990s which created the semi-autonomous hospital and community trusts have implications about the ownership of, and access to, medical postgraduate centres. This may result in rental charges for premises used for some day-release courses.

Most of these items are the direct responsibility of others (for example, the trainer deals with the salary and car allowance of the registrar). The following generalizations indicate who is *usually* responsible for what (after Garrett, 1992).

Regional postgraduate council

Reorganization of provision for postgraduate education has resulted in deans becoming fundholders for the total postgraduate training budget including vocational training and CME (NHS Management Executive, 1991). They are responsible for:

- salaries (of course organizers, the regional and associate directors and regional office staff. They are also responsible for a proportion of the salaries of all doctors in hospital training grades)
- course expenses (for special events for trainers and trainees, e.g. residential courses organized at regional level, drawing on section 63 funds)
- equipment and staffing of regional office facilities, and obtaining special equipment which may be available on loan from central sources
- expenses (e.g. for travel to committee and regional meetings)
- the registrar's salary and car allowance are paid by the trainer as the employer. The trainer is reimbursed for this and receives the trainer's grant through the usual channel of payment for GPs.

The hospital trust

The postgraduate clinical tutor has an executive function here (NHS Management Executive, 1991). He is directly responsible to the postgraduate dean for ensuring that there are educational facilities and proper standards of in-service training. The hospital provides half of the salary of SHO trainees and is responsible for their study leave, provides medical postgraduate centre facilities and employs the postgraduate centre secretary.

Section 63

This is a statutory fund administered in England and Wales by the regional director's office for the payment of travel and subsistence expenses of those who are involved in vocational training: trainees, trainers and course organizers. Funding is limited. A proportion of expenses will be reimbursed on request, and at the end of the financial year any residual funds will be distributed as a supplement. In Northern Ireland its equivalent is the extended study leave budget administered by the Central Services Agency.

Day-release course budget

This is often a notional or indicative budget, with all reasonable recurring expenses underwritten and administered by the regional office. In such cases each day-release course is given an annual figure as a guideline. Some course organizers have to work within strict budgetary limits. A typical figure for a day-release course is about £2000 annually. Some regions apply a limit of about £200 to any single-day event, unless there is a special case to be made and alternative funding is available as well. A typical speaker's fee is in the region of £55 to £65 per session. Some may not require payment if education of doctors is part of their remit (e.g. the police drug squad education officer).

Commercial sponsorship

Representatives of the pharmaceutical industry are often keen to obtain access to groups of trainees through the day-release course. They have a code of practice which governs any financial transactions involved. These might include sponsorship of additional expenses, e.g. catering for a seminar or other special event, or the purchase of an educational resource such as teaching materials (videos, books etc.). There may be regional policy on such matters in addition to the guidelines of ethical practice. It is important that the course organizer, as a role model for the trainees, maintains a high standard of conduct in this respect. Relations with the pharmaceutical industry and how to deal with company representatives may be a useful discussion topic for the curriculum.

'Slush' fund

Needless to say, no course organizer has one, but if he had it might be used as petty cash for buying coffee for the day-release course, providing interim payments to cover delays in section 63 reimbursement, and making occasional small purchases such as books. Sponsorship donations from pharmaceutical companies are sometimes used for such purposes. Accountability is important and it is advisable to maintain a petty cash ledger. Course organizers' legitimate out-of-pocket expenses, e.g. buying blank video tapes for teaching purposes, may be reimbursed directly from the regional office. If in doubt consult the regional director.

The course organizer's personal finances

The finances of medical practice are complicated. Being a course organizer may add a further complexity. Your salary as course organizer will come to you net of tax at basic rate, pension fund and national insurance contribution (NIC). Your accountant will want to know the figures. They will affect the tax situation and the rate of deduction for NIC from your GP income since this will already have been partly paid by the deductions from your course organizer pay. As a result the accountant will probably arrange for deferral of NI payments. This has two consequences: a level of NIC deductions from your monthly practice income which differs from those of your partners, and a large bill once a year for the balance of NI contributions.

Being a course organizer makes demands on time, energy and availability for practice work. Before taking up the course organizer post, it is essential to clarify with your partners how these competing interests will be reconciled. Most practices have an agreement covering issues relating to employment outside the practice. Many course organizers run into difficulties with their partners through misunderstandings arising from this.

Guidelines

To sum up, you should:

- know your regional structure and who is responsible for what

- watch your budget margin, especially towards the financial year end
- make sure your invited resource persons are paid promptly
- review with your secretary the procedures she follows
- keep a clear record of approved expenses and claim promptly
- be financially accountable; keep a petty cash book
- be a good role model for trainees in your relations with pharmaceutical represent-atives, especially where sponsorship is concerned
- keep your partners happy and do not 'steal' time from them
- have a clear agreement about use of locums and other ways of covering for neces-sary absence
- refer issues of uncertainty to the regional director
- pay your accountant and spare your coronaries!

Visitations

In the UK co-ordination of vocational training, maintenance of standards and en-forcement of regulations are carried out through a system of visitations. This system has features of both peer review and formative assessment of the various strata of vocational training.

1 All training practices are visited by representatives of the region before approval, and periodically for reapproval.
2 All day-release courses may be visited by the regional director or his deputy at any time, informally.
3 All hospital training posts are visited by delegates of the respective colleges, specialty ruling bodies or Joint Committee.
4 All regions are visited by the Joint Committee to assess the total work of the region in general practice vocational training.

Course organizers play a large part in these proceedings and may be called upon to take part in panels of visitors for any of the above purposes. For matters relating to hospital posts and liaison with consultants, *see* Chapter 12.

The training practice visit

This is a delicate and demanding task, especially if you are conducting a visit on your own patch. Are you present:

- on peer visitation as an equal?
- as a 'friend of the trainer' with an advocacy role?

1	Trainer is well informed about the teaching role	0	5
2	Trainer shows evidence of continued development of his or her teaching skills	0	5
3	Trainer has a discernible philosophy of education and overall aims	0	5
4	Trainer uses an adequate range of educational techniques	0	5
5	Trainer produced an adequate curriculum for teaching	0	5
6	Trainer gives adequate protected time for teaching	0	5
7	Training practice fosters interdisciplinary co-operation	0	5
8	Training practice shows evidence of audit involving the trainee	0	5
9	Practice maintains appropriate quality of records	0	5
10	Practice library adequate and well organized	0	5
11	Facilities for registrar adequate	0	5
12	Practice premises adequate	0	5

Figure 15.3 Template for recording a training practice visit.

- as an independent observer?
- as a representative of the regional director?

It is important to clarify for yourself in advance which one (or more) of these roles you are expected to adopt, and to remind yourself throughout the proceedings of your role and function. Ask the regional director, and others experienced in practice visitation, to brief you about the region's tradition of practice and the aims of the exercise. Particular aims will include ensuring compliance with the JCPTGP and regional criteria; general aims will include gaining an overview of the practice, assessing the educational competence of the trainer, inspecting the premises and provision for the trainee, and enquiring about the registrar's satisfaction.

In the role of 'friend of the trainer' it may be legitimate to brief him or her before the visit, help to identify problems (and rectify them in advance), and even conduct a mock visit. A template for assessment is shown in Figure 15.3.

The report

In compiling the report on the visit, the principles of formative assessment should be borne in mind, along with 'Pendleton's Rules'.

1 Note the trainer's own reflections on his or her strengths and weaknesses, and those of the practice.

2 State what is done well.

3 Adopt the perspective of 'how far the training practice has come' rather than that of 'where it is at', especially with regard to applying the criteria.

4 Formulate a positive critique of the training offered by this practice, offering constructive suggestions to accompany any critical observation.

5 Be clear and realistic in the summary and recommendations.

6 The report is not a decision but a recommendation.

The report on the visit is sent to the regional director as executive officer of the trainer selection committee. There may be an uncomfortable summative element in addition to the formative process of visitation. In cases of difficulty there is likely to be conflict, and it is important to be aware of the terms of reference and appeals procedure. Course organizers who are inexperienced in visitation should 'serve their time' as observers or junior members before allowing themselves to be delegated a leading role in visiting.

The minimum educational criteria for training practices are listed in Part 6.

The Joint Committee visit (JCPTGP)

Before taking part in, or being subjected to, a Joint Committee visit it is important to explore the structure and functions of this body, through reading their booklets (JCPTGP, 1992a,b). The Joint Committee on Postgraduate Training for General Practice is the ruling body of vocational training recognized by statute, and the competent authority for supervision of training under the European Directive. It is drawn mainly from the Royal College of General Practitioners and the General Medical Services Committee (related to the British Medical Association) but there are also representatives from the universities, the Department of Health, the Association of Course Organizers, the armed forces and clinical tutors.

Its brief is to ensure consistent application of the statutes – the National Health Service (Vocational Training) Regulations (1997) and the equivalents in Scotland and Northern Ireland – and to monitor all training arrangements. It is the certifying body which issues the certificates necessary for appointment as a principal in general practice.

There is a regular two-yearly cycle of visits to regional training schemes and those of the armed forces. This is resourced by a panel of about 70 visitors, most of whom are regional or associate directors or course organizers. Each visit is carried out by three members of the panel and lasts three days. Components of individual schemes are inspected. The general pattern is:

- a visit to about 10 training practices, usually from one sector of the region. In each one they will wish to interview the trainer, the practice manager and the registrar
- a visit to the day-release course which relates to those practices, interviewing the course organizer(s)

- a private session with the trainees collectively
- a meeting with the region's course organizers collectively
- a meeting with the hospital chief executive, clinical tutors and consultants collectively or individually
- private meetings with the dean, regional and associate directors
- private time for deliberation and preparation of their feedback report to a final meeting of officers of the regional council. This will form the basis of the eventual report to the JCPTGP.

The practical arrangements are usually in the hands of the regional director but he may delegate this to an associate director or course organizer.

A copy of the report is sent to the dean and regional director, who is expected to report its findings to the general practice committee and develop plans for implementing any formal recommendations.

At the next visit to the region the visitors will be expected to enquire about progress with the recommendations. Failure to comply with formal recommendations can result in withdrawal of recognition of the region's training scheme. Various Joint Committee publications (JCPTGP, 1992a,b, 1997) summarize its terms of reference, policies and methods. They describe the aims of the visit under 12 headings.

1 To report on the extent of the region's implementation of criteria for approval of trainers and if they follow Joint Committee recommendations.
2 To review standards of vocational training and note desirable features.
3 To identify districts providing the required standard.
4 To make recommendations to the region for improvement.
5 To identify local conditions hampering full implementation of Joint Committee policies and to provide encouragement and help.
6 To identify national and regional policies which are detrimental to vocational training so that the Joint Committee can inform its constituent bodies.
7 To note the availability of part-time training.
8 To assess the provision of counselling for trainees.
9 To encourage the regional director, course organizers and trainers to audit their work.
10 To encourage innovation and improvement in standards and to disseminate examples of good practice.
11 To foster goodwill between the Joint Committee and the region; to show trainees that there is a body which is concerned about their standards of provision.
12 To promote peer assessment and quality in care and teaching.

A full-scale Joint Committee visit can be gruelling for all concerned. At the same time it is important to note the positive intentions of the items on the list: to enable, advise, help, disseminate information.

Figure 15.4 shows a template designed for the occasional course organizer who is elected to organize the visit (after Terry, 1991).

1 *What are they looking for?*
Regional educational policy aims achieved.
Regional criteria for appointment/re-appointment of trainers being observed.
Evidence of what is being done well locally in:
  • training practices
  • hospital training posts
  • day-release courses
  • trainers' workshops.
Educational developments, especially in assessment and audit.
Evidence of problem areas and strains.
Recommendations of previous visitors implemented.

2 *Programme of the visit*
Whom will they meet? (Dean, regional director and associates, chairman of the general practice committee, course organizers, selected training practices, the clinical tutor and selected consultants, trainees (including SHOs) and administrative staff.)
Work out times, including transit times; will it work?
Do not overload it; leave short spaces between tasks.
Consider a 'dry run' with regional directors and target practices.
Note: for the three days' duration you are totally committed. Arrange time out of the practice.

3 *Prepare material*
Work out the itinerary and timetable
Consider preparing videos of practice visits, the day-release course in action, or trainee tutorials with trainers.
Read annual reports of day-release courses and practices.
Look up reports of previous visits.

4 *During the visit*
Make sure they are met and welcomed by regional office-bearers.
Begin with briefing, giving a profile of the region, the day-release courses and training practices.
Ensure that the practices know the timetable.
Make sure the visitors are properly hosted and accommodated (remember Maslow?), with time and facilities for working together privately at the end of the day.
Have a working dinner in the middle. The visitors want to mingle and meet everybody.
Each evening, take time to review the day with a colleague and check arrangements for next day.
Do not pack too much into last day; do allow time for feedback, end early to minimize battle fatigue, and debrief the main participants after visitors' departure: what has been learned?

Figure 15.4 Planning for a joint committee visit to a district scheme.

The Association of Course Organizers*

Origins

Three-year vocational training schemes began to gain momentum during the late 1960s. In 1972, the role of the course organizer (as a trainer with special responsibilities) was recognized in the 'Red Book'. By the mid-1970s most district general hospitals had a vocational training scheme including a day or half-day release course run by a course organizer. In 1974, Paul Freeling ran a 'modular' course – the Nuffield course – for course organizers. This had a far-reaching influence on the ethos and methods of vocational training. Even now, most course organizers are either graduates of that course themselves or have been heavily influenced by somebody who was.

Following the Nuffield course there were various shorter training events for course organizers, for instance at the University of Warwick (by David Clegg) and through the MSD Foundation (by Marshall Marinker). In 1980, Michael Whitfield and Roddy Hughes from Bristol conducted a national survey of the work of course organizers, and the results were discussed at a one-day conference in 1981. Following this conference an unsuccessful attempt was made to form a national association of course organizers. By then vocational training was mandatory and the workload of course organizers had become much greater and more complex than anyone had envisaged 10 years previously. This resulted in what Jamie Bahrami in 1985 described as *'a volcano of resentment and frustration which, until the formation of the Association of Course Organizers, had been little appreciated by the profession'*.

Perhaps even more widespread than this feeling of resentment was the uncertainty and isolation felt by course organizers, many of whom were, by the early 1980s, second-generation course organizers. When I visited 34 schemes in 1984 to do research into small group work on the release course, I was forcibly struck by how anxious course organizers were to obtain feedback about their performance in relation to others.

It was in this climate of professional isolation that the Association of Course Organizers was finally formed in 1984. The one advantage of the trainer status of course organizers was that, in theory, unlimited numbers could be appointed. Many regions had succeeded in appointing several course organizers to each scheme thus alleviating both the isolation and the heavy workload. In other regions, course organizers were not convinced of the need for a national association. Had it not been for the energy and determination of Jamie Bahrami of Yorkshire Region it is most unlikely that the Association would have got off the ground.

*Author's note: I am indebted to Dr Paul Sackin for this account of the history of the ACO

Aims

The first conference of the Association in 1985 agreed overwhelmingly that the primary aim of the ACO was 'educational' rather than 'political'. This decision rapidly helped to persuade most course organizers to become members. The broad aims of the ACO, as stated in the constitution, still hold:

- to explore and develop the role and responsibilities of course organizers
- to plan and implement regular educational opportunities for course organizers
- to collect and provide information on all matters relating to the work of course organizers
- to represent course organizers on appropriate local and national representative bodies.

Achievements

The achievements of the Association have been impressive by any standards.

1 *The Journal of the Association of Course Organizers* ran from Autumn 1985 to Spring 1990, being issued three times a year. Under the editorship of Declan Dwyer, the journal was from the start a major influence on postgraduate education for general practice. It provided a forum for course organizers (and others) to share and develop ideas. Its uniquely informal style allowed well-researched but eminently readable papers to sit comfortably alongside humour, news and short descriptions of new ideas in training. The journal was supported by Upjohn. When their sponsorship ended, the journal was reborn as *Postgraduate Education for General Practice*, launched in 1990 by Radcliffe Medical Press. This journal continued to appear three times a year under Declan Dwyer's energetic editorship. Initially there was some concern that the new journal would be too 'academic' and less relevant to course organizers, but every effort has been made to combine the values of the old journal with the desire for a slightly broader appeal and for more rigorously refereed main papers. The growing realization that we share common concerns with other GP educators – academic staff in university departments of general practice and postgraduate (CME) tutors – led to further developments. Its title was changed to *Education for General Practice*. Editions are now produced four times per year, which makes it eligible for citation in international indexing and abstracting works. It has a growing international reputation with uptake and contributions from far beyond these shores.
2 *Conferences and courses*. The Association of Course Organizers has run annual conferences at Ripon since 1985. These have gradually become less structured as members feel more confident about running their own groups. The conferences have enormously enhanced the 'family' atmosphere of the Association, with plenty of opportunity for informal discussion and humour. AGMs have invariably been

lively and often controversial. I cannot recall meeting anyone leaving Ripon other than refreshed and full of new ideas to try out.

The Association sponsors an annual course of new course organizers at Cumberland Lodge. In the early years attempts were made to run other national courses, in particular on small group leadership. Excellent as many of these were, they were not well supported. In more recent years the ACO has been delighted to be associated with regular courses on small group work run by Mary Davis and Peter Jenkins.

3 *Assessment of trainees.* The journal and conferences have contributed enormously to the development of all aspects of vocational training. Assessment has been a particular feature, with the publication in 1988 of an influential ACO working party report – *Trainee centred assessment.* Although the ACO has always favoured formative assessment it has had regular dialogue on examination matters with the Royal College of General Practitioners and the JCPTGP. Since 1990 the ACO has had representation on the examination board of the College, an acknowledgement by the College of the important contribution of course organizers to assessment. The Association also made representations to the Joint Committee on the introduction of the summative assessment procedure.

4 *Liaison with other bodies.* Over the years the RCGP has sought the views of the ACO on a variety of issues. The ACO is represented on CAOGP, the umbrella group of GP academic bodies convened by the College. These closer links have helped the College to appreciate fully the importance of course organizers and this has led to a great deal of help and support in the quest for proper recognition by government. The Association also has a representative on the Joint Committee. The ACO worked closely with the GMSC in the protracted, but ultimately successful, attempts to improve the remuneration of course organizers. The ACO representatives have, on occasions, been able to participate in direct negotiations with the Department of Health.

5 *Course organizer's remuneration.* Successive secretaries of the Association, with the help of many other members, campaigned hard to take course organizers' pay out of target net remuneration and to negotiate for pay on the consultant scale. This effort bore fruit with an agreement reached with the Department of Health in 1992, just hours before the majority of course organizers were due to submit their resignations. The lengthy negotiations had a number of useful spin-offs. For example, the course organizers' job description drawn up by Dr Donald Fairclough and colleagues in 1985, and the workload study by Dr Antony Lewis in the same year, led to important debates about the whole nature of vocational training.

6 *ACO fellowships.* Since 1990, the Association has offered an annual Fellowship to support research and development work relevant to the aims of the Association. The contributions of the various Fellowship holders – Drs Roger Neighbour, Oliver Samuel, Antony Lewis, Patrick McEvoy and Jonathan Silverman – have been extremely impressive and have done a great deal to enhance many aspects of vocational training. The ACO has also sponsored doctors from Africa to attend the Ripon conference.

7 *ACO and the press.* The Association has enjoyed an extremely open relationship with the 'popular' medical press, with the secretary acting as press officer. This has not always been without controversy but overall the relationship has been very successful. It has led to widespread coverage of course organizing matters, and to a readiness by reporters to approach the ACO for background information on all aspects of training for general practice.

The future

These tangible achievements are impressive, but perhaps the most important aspect of the ACO is the ethos it has established. It combines enthusiasm, openness and humour, especially with regard to group skills and practical new ideas. These characteristics pervade everything that the ACO has done and I feel sure that they will remain. I hope that the future will bring even closer links between the ACO and Association of GP Tutors. If the proposals of the RCGP are accepted (and it seems reasonable to expect that eventually they will be) these roles will become much less distinct and both course organizers and GP tutors will become associate directors. The ACO will have an enormous amount to contribute to such generic GP postgraduate educators. I believe that this development would also help the progress of *Education for General Practice*, which is now firmly established as the only journal of education for general practice independent of commercial sponsorship and advertising.

Attempts have been made through the ACO to forge links between course organizers and their opposite numbers abroad. Members of the ACO have been involved in developing general practice training programmes in central and eastern Europe and the Middle East. I expect this trend to continue in the future, particularly with our European partners.

During most of the ACO's existence, general practice has been developing in an exciting way and has attracted the very best medical graduates. The last few years have seen this atmosphere change and many young doctors are, at best, uncertain about entertaining a career in general practice. This situation presents a challenge to many young people and organizations. I have little doubt that course organizers and the ACO will rise to this challenge, giving back to the trainees (and others) some of the lost enthusiasm.

In this materialistic age, course organizers may ask what joining the ACO will give them. In material terms, they may have to make do with a reduced subscription to the journal, an introductory information pack and a free copy of this Handbook, but they will gain the immeasurable benefits of belonging to as friendly and stimulating a club as any I know.

16

Vocational training database

Introduction

A recurring theme in this book has been to emphasize the diversity of tasks, structures and working practices affecting course organizing in different parts of the United Kingdom and Ireland. This is further reflected in the variety of organizations, regulations and resources that you may encounter in reality or in the course of your reading. The survey in Part 1 identified the need for a vade-mecum, a database to meet recurring or occasional information needs. Much information of this kind is scattered throughout the various chapters; other factual matters are gathered together in this section. Our information needs differ and require constant updating, but here are some suggestions about where to begin.

Organizations related to vocational training

ACO (Association of Course Organizers)

Contact:	Mrs Allyson Horner (Administrator) c/o Cleveland GP Scheme Grey Towers Court Stokesley Road Nanthorpe Middlesbrough TS7 0PN
Tel:	01642 304151
Fax:	01642 304157
Website:	*http://www.aco.org.uk*
Membership:	open to all course organizers in the UK.

Each region elects one representative to Executive Council. The (Irish) National Association of Programme Directors sends one representative who is a non-voting participant. For full details of the history and activities of the ACO, see Chapter 15.

Publication:	*Education for General Practice* (Published quarterly by Radcliffe Medical Press, Oxford)
Editor:	Dr Declan Dwyer 167 North Road West Plymouth PL1 5BZ
Tel:	01752 662780
Fax:	01752 254541

AMEE (Association for Medical Education in Europe)

Contact:	Pat Lilley Centre for Medical Education Tay Park 484 Perth Road Dundee DD2 1LR
Tel:	01382 631967
Fax:	01382 645748
e-mail:	*p.m.lilley@dundee.ac.uk*
Membership:	individual and corporate. Approx 700 members. Individual membership fee is £38.
Aim:	to promote expertise in medical education.

Its priorities are the study of education in medicine and health care professions and to foster communication among the teachers. It links with national associations of medical education in Europe and worldwide through the World Federation for Medical Education.

Publication:	*Medical Teacher* (Carfax).

Published six times per year, it is the official journal of the AMEE and appears in English. AMEE also publishes guides on key educational matters.

ASGPAB (Armed Services General Practice Approval Board)

Contact: Colonel John Dickinson (Secretary)
                Fort Blockhouse
                Gosport
                Hants PO12 2AB

Tel: 01705 765667

Fax: 01705 765667

The ASGPAB is the equivalent of a regional office and is responsible for inspecting all service practices and approved hospital posts. The board consists of an independent chairman appointed by the Secretary of State, two representatives of the RCGP and one from the Department of Health, civilian consultants in general practice to each service, three service advisers in general practice, and a secretary appointed by the Surgeon General.

ASME (Association for the Study of Medical Education)

Contact: Juliet Young (Administrator)
                The Lister Institute
                11 Hill Square
                Edinburgh EH8 9DR

Tel: 0131 662 1161

Fax: 0131 662 1171

e-mail: *info@asme.org.uk*

Website: *http://www.asme.org.uk*

Membership: mostly doctors involved in teaching/learning in the field of medical education at all levels and across all the specialties.

Aim: to promote expertise in medical education.

Publishes various papers and reports on medical education. Meets four to six times per year on topics related to medical education.

Publication: *Medical Education* (Blackwell Science)

AUDGP (Association of University Departments of General Practice)

Contact: Dr John Campbell (Secretary)
Dept of General Practice
UMDS
5 Lambeth Walk
London SE11 6ST

Tel: 0171 735 8881

Fax: 0171 793 7232

e-mail: *j.campbell@umds.ac.uk*

Aim: to promote the development of general practice as a university discipline.

Membership: members of academic departments of general practice in the UK.

The Balint Society

Contact: Dr David Watt (Secretary)
Tollgate Health Centre
220 Tollgate Road
London E6 4JS

Tel: 0171 445 7709

Fax: 0171 445 7715

Membership: open to all GPs who have completed one year in a Balint group. Associate membership is open to anyone involved in health care.

The Society was founded in 1969 to promote learning and to continue the research into the understanding of the doctor/patient relationship which was the unique legacy of Michael and Enid Balint. Regular meetings and conferences, including the bi-annual International Balint Conference, are organized by the International Balint Federation.

Publication: *Journal of the Balint Society*

Editor: Dr Philip Hopkins, FRCGP
249 Haverstock Hill
London NW3 4PS

Tel: 0171 431 6826

BPMF (British Postgraduate Medical Federation)

A coalition of the four London regions. It ceased to function in 1996. *See* SLOVTS.

British Library

Address:	The British Library
	Boston Spa
	Wetherby
	West Yorkshire LS23 7BQ
Tel:	01937 546000
Website:	*http://www.bl.uk*

The Document Supply Centre at the above address is normally accessed through the local medical library. Individuals can use their services directly on a fee-paying basis. On-line searches can be commissioned through its Health Care Information Service (Tel: 0171 412 7477).

The British Library is a complex national institution which operates from a number of different locations. Its facilities are described in great detail on its website. The on-line catalogue can be accessed on http://opac97.bl.uk.

CAIPE (UK Centre for the Advancement of Inter-Professional Education)

Contact:	Lyn Smith (Director)
	344 Gray's Inn Road
	London WC1X 8BP
Tel:	0171 278 1083
Fax:	0171 278 6604
Aims:	to improve quality in health care through promoting interprofessional collaboration, respecting the contribution of each profession and encouraging professionals to learn with, from and about each other.
Publication:	*Journal of Interprofessional Care* (Carfax).

CAOGP (Conference of Academic Organizations in General Practice)

Chairman: Professor Denis Pereira-Gray

Contact: Francesca Ohene-Djan (Administrator)
               RCGP
               11 Princes Gate
               London SW7 1PU

Tel: 0171 381 3232

Fax: 0171 225 3047

e-mail: *info@rcgp.org.uk*

Established in 1989, this standing committee is composed of a representative of each of the organizations that contribute to education for general practice – heads of university departments of general practice, RCGP, AUDGP, JCPTGP, COGPED, ACO, NAGPT and the General Practice Research Framework of the MRC. It provides a forum for examining the educational implications of changes in public policy, legislation and service conditions in academic general practice; disseminating information of mutual interest to the contributing organizations and, particularly, in giving expression to the concerns of GP academics in promoting research, development and teaching.

Centre for Evidence-based Medicine

Director: Professor David Sackett

Contact: Olive Goddard (Centre Co-ordinator)
               Centre for Evidence-based Medicine
               Nuffield Department of Clinical Medicine
               The John Radcliffe
               Headington
               Oxford OX3 9DU

Tel: 01865 221321

Fax: 01865 222901

e-mail: *oliveg@cebm.jr2.ox.ac.uk*

Website: *http://cebm.jr2.ox.ac.uk*

Cochrane Collaboration

Address: UK Cochrane Centre
               Summertown Pavilion
               Middle Way
               Oxford OX2 7LG

Tel:	01865 516300
Fax:	01865 516311
e-mail:	*cochrane@vax.ox.ac.uk*
Website:	*www.cochrane.co.uk*

Named after Archie Cochrane, this is a worldwide network of centres devoted to the production of evidence-based databases collating the findings of controlled trials published in medical journals.

The Cochrane Library consists of a number of specialized databases available on disk or CD-ROM on annual subscription and regularly updated:

- The Cochrane Database of Systematic Reviews (CDSR)
- The Database of Abstracts of Reviews of Effectiveness (DARE)
- The Cochrane Controlled Trials Register (CCTR)
- The Cochrane Review of Methodology Database (CRMD)
- The Cochrane Pregnancy and Childbirth Database.

Further information may be accessed on:

http://hiru.mcmaster.ca/cochrane/.

COGPED (Conference of General Practice Education Directors)

Contact:	Anne Mochrie (Business Manager) 33 Millman Street London WC1N 3EJ
Tel:	0171 692 3197
Fax:	0171 404 2930
e-mail:	*copmed@tpmde.ac.uk*
Membership:	Regional Directors of Postgraduate Education for General Practice, a representative of the Directors in the Armed Forces and the Chairman of COPMED.

By contrast with CRAGPIE, which it replaces, it has a UK-wide remit as a forum for developing initiatives and a consensus view on the management of postgraduate general practice education. It liaises closely with the UK Conference of Regional Advisers in General Practice.

COPMED (Committee of Postgraduate Medical Deans)

| Contact: | Anne Mochrie (Business Manager)
33 Millman Street
London WC1N 3EJ |

Tel: 0171 692 3197

Fax: 0171 404 2930

e-mail: *copmed@tpmde.ac.uk*

Membership: all Postgraduate Medical Deans

Formed in 1997 by the fusion of two bodies – COPMED and The UK Conference (The Conference of Postgraduate Medical Deans and Directors of Postgraduate Medical Education of Universities of the United Kingdom (UKRA)). Its remit is to share good practice in all matters relating to medical education, training and welfare of junior doctors; to advise government, universities, NHS Executive and commissioning agencies on all matters relating to postgraduate and continuing medical education; to liaise with other relevant bodies (Council of Deans of Medical Schools, GMC, Royal Colleges etc.); to promote research, development, multidisciplinary learning and liaise with European counterparts.

CRAGPIE (Committee of Regional Advisers in General Practice in England)

This body has been subsumed into the new Committee of General Practice Education Directors (COGPED) which has a remit for the whole UK (*see* COGPED).

Dundee University Centre for Medical Education

Contact: Mrs Sue Roff
                Tay Park House
                484 Perth Road
                Dundee DD2 1LR

Tel: 01382 631968

Fax: 01382 645748

Established in 1977 to promote the improvement of postgraduate and continuing medical education, its key activities include research and teaching in medical education and the development of distance learning. It offers postgraduate qualifications in medical education (certificate, diploma, master's degree and PhD), directly or by distance learning, as well as short courses and workshops. Vocational training contributions include assessment (such as OSCE) and the development of learning resources.

EGPRW (European General Practice Research Workshop)

A sub-division of the European Society of General Practice/Family Medicine. May be contacted through EURACT.

EURACT (European Academy of Teachers in General Practice)

Contact: Dr Justin Allen (UK representative)
               Countesthorpe Health Centre
               Central Street
               Countesthorpe
               Leicester LE8 3QJ

Tel: 0116 277 6336

Fax: 0116 278 0851

e-mail: *justina@pipex.dial.com*

Membership: all teachers of general practice in the WONCA (World Organization
               of National Colleges, Academics and Academic Associations of
               GPs and Family Physicians) European region on payment of fee
               (ECU 40, approx £30). Membership is subject to acceptance of
               nomination by the Council of the Academy.

The history of EURACT can be traced back to the first Leeuwenhorst Group in 1974.
Its successor, the New Leeuwenhorst Group, was formed in 1982. The Academy provides resources, meetings and support for teachers of general practice. It is a constituent of the European Society of General Practice/Family Medicine in conjunction
with EGPRW and WONCA-Europe. They jointly support the *European Journal of General Practice* (Mediselect Publishing, PO Box 28091, 3828 ZH Hoogland, Netherlands;
Tel: 00 31 33 808020; Fax: 00 31 33 805881).

European Society of General Practice/Family Medicine

Formed in 1995 at a conference in Strasbourg through the amalgamation of WONCA-
Europe and SIMG. It has three sub-divisions:

1 EURACT – European Academy of Teachers in General Practice
2 EGPRW – European GP Research Workshop
3 EQUIP – European Quality In Practice Network.

Publication: *The European Journal of General Practice Quarterly*

Address: Mediselect Publishing
               PO Box 28091
               3828 ZH Hoogland
               Netherlands

Tel: 00 31 33 808020

Fax: 00 31 33 805881

Faculty of Family Planning and Reproductive Health Care

Contact: The Membership and Training Secretary
27 Sussex Place
Regent's Park
London NW1 4RG

Tel: 0171 723 3175

Fax: 0171 723 0575

A faculty of the Royal College of Obstetricians and Gynaecologists established in 1993 by merging the National Association of Family Planning Doctors and the Joint Committee on Contraception.

The Faculty grants diplomas, certificates and equivalent recognition of specialist knowledge and skills in family planning and reproductive health care. It promotes conferences and lectures and provides an advisory service.

Publication: *The British Journal of Family Planning* (published quarterly)

Qualifications: MFFP – Membership of the Faculty of Family Planning
DFFP – Diploma of the Faculty of Family Planning

GMSC (General Medical Services Committee)

Address: GMSC
BMA House
Tavistock Square
London WC1H 9JP

Tel: 0171 387 4499

Fax: 0171 383 6400

Membership: elected representatives of Local Medical Committees (LMCs).

Established under the auspices of the BMA, it represents all GPs in the UK irrespective of BMA membership. Its particular remit is to negotiate with the Department of Health, regional offices of the NHS and purchasing authorities about the terms and conditions of service for GPs. Although not primarily an educational body it has an Education and Training Sub-Committee. Representatives of the GMSC sit on Postgraduate Councils. It was jointly responsible with the RCGP for setting up the Joint Committee (JCPTGP).

Whereas the RCGP represents the academic/educational wing of general practice, the GMSC complements this by representing the service aspect.

ICGP (Irish College of General Practitioners)

Contact:	The Secretary 4–5 Lincoln Place Dublin 2
Tel:	003531 6763705
Fax:	003531 6765850
e-mail:	*info@icgp.ie*
Website:	*http://indigo.ie/~ icgp/index.html*
Membership:	by examination (MICGP)

Founded in 1984, it is recognized by the Medical Council of Ireland and the Irish government as the representative academic and certifying body for the specialty of general practice. It is organized on a county-based faculty structure.

It is responsible for standards of vocational training in the Republic of Ireland through the Committee for Visiting and Approving Training Programmes. This is a sub-committee of the Board of Censors. Major visits to all programmes take place every five years.

Joint Centre for Education in Medicine

Director:	Professor Janet Grant
Contact:	Sarah Flood (Project Secretary) 33 Millman Street London WC1N 3EJ
Tel:	0171 692 3145
Fax:	0171 692 3109
e-mail:	*j.centre@ppmde.ac.uk*
Aim:	to improve the quality of medical education through action research involving those who provide, manage and receive postgraduate medical education. It undertakes an extensive programme of research, projects and publishing.

JCPTGP (Joint Committee on Postgraduate Training for General Practice)

Address: 14 Princes Gate
                  London SW7 1PU

Tel: 0171 581 3232

Fax: 0171 589 5047

e-mail: *info@rcgp.org.uk*

In 1974, the RCGP and the GMSC set up a special Committee for Postgraduate Training. In 1975 it broadened its membership and became the JCPTGP. Its 25 members are drawn from: the RCGP (seven, including one trainee); the GMSC (seven, including one trainee); COGPED (three); the Joint Consultants Committee (three); and the ACO, ASGPAB, AUDGP, COPMED and NACT (one each). Meetings are attended by observers from the Department of Health and Councils for Postgraduate Medical Education. The secretariat consists of an administrative secretary, two joint honorary secretaries, one administrative secretary, and a medical adviser with special responsibility for certification. The Committee:

- advises professional and educational bodies on standards for postgraduate training for general practice
- monitors regional training arrangements and recognizes programmes
- performs statutory functions specified in NHS (VT) Regulation 1997
- is the Responsible Authority for certification for general practice under the European Directive (for further details *see* Chapter 15).

King's Fund – King Edward's Hospital Fund for London

Contact: Information Officer
                  11–13 Cavendish Square
                  London W1M 0AN

Tel: 0171 307 2585

Fax: 0171 307 2805

e-mail: *a.forbes@kehf.org.uk*

King Edward's Hospital Fund for London was founded in 1897. It seeks to stimulate good practice and innovation in all aspects of health care and management through research and development, education, policy analysis and funding. It does not fund basic scientific or clinical research. Its main activities include making grants to London hospitals (via the Jubilee Project), and assessing and promoting the quality of health care in the inner city, through the London Primary Care programme; analysis of public health policy through conferences, working parties and publications; supporting innovation in NHS-related organizations.

The King's Fund College was founded in 1968 to raise standards of management in health care.

NACT (National Association of Clinical Tutors)

Contact:	The Secretary 12 Chandos Street London W1M 9DE
Tel:	0171 290 3930
Fax:	0171 290 3932
e-mail:	*nact@globalnet.co.uk*
Membership:	open to clinical tutors who have been appointed by universities.

NACT was formed in 1969 to assist clinical tutors in their role as co-ordinators of medical education at district hospital level. Activities include courses for the training and continuing professional development of clinical tutors. National meetings take place twice yearly.

Publications:	*Directory of Postgraduate Medical Centres* *NACT Training Package*

NAGPT (UK) (National Association of GP Tutors (UK))

Contact:	Dr K Kotegaonkar (Chairman) The Surgery 17 Spring Lane Radcliffe Manchester M26 2TQ
Tel:	0161 723 2145
Fax:	0161 723 2145
Membership:	any GP tutor or GP carrying out an equivalent function. At present there are about 350 members.
Aim:	'Towards wisdom and health'

Objectives:

To support its members by:

1 providing a platform for educational development
2 addressing their learning needs
3 creating an educational network
4 representing the interests of GP tutors
5 establishing a national identity for GP tutors.

Publications: Participates in *Education for General Practice*, provides a *Directory of GP Tutors* and aims to produce a quarterly bulletin through *Update*.

It organizes one national conference annually and is planning an annual training conference and a Millenium conference.

NAPD (National Association of Programme Directors)

Contact: Mrs Annette Elebert
c/o Irish College of General Practitioners
4–5 Lincoln Place
Dublin 2

Tel: 003531 6763705

Fax: 003531 6765850

e-mail: *info@icgp.ie*

Membership: all Programme Directors and Assistant Directors from the 10 training programmes in Ireland.

Meets twice yearly. Principal aim is to meet the educational needs of members. Equivalent to the Association of Course Organizers in the UK. Training programmes in the Republic of Ireland are similar to those in the UK – two years in hospital attachments, one year in a training practice. There is a total national intake of 54 trainees per year to the 10 schemes. One scheme (Sligo) runs a four-year course which includes one year in community health.

Network of Community Oriented Educational Institutions for Health Sciences

Contact: Pauline Vluggen
Network Secretariat
PO Box 616
6200 MD Maastricht
Netherlands

Tel:	00 31 43 388 1522
Fax:	00 31 43 367 0708
e-mail:	*g.majoor@bibfdg.unimas.nl*

Founded in 1979 with a network of over 240 members (individual and institutions) worldwide, in official relation with WHO and the United Nations.

Its main focus is on innovation, examining the needs for change and planning, implementation and evaluation especially through education and training of health workers.

Publication:	*Education for Health: change in training and practice* (Carfax)
Address:	Professor Charles Engel (Editor) Centre for Higher Education Studies Institute of Education University of London 55–59 Gordon Square London WC1H 0NT
Tel:	0171 612 6363

NICPMDE (Northern Ireland Council for Postgraduate Medical and Dental Education)

Contact:	Dr J McCluggage (Dean of Postgraduate Medicine) 5 Annadale Avenue Belfast BT7 3JH
Tel:	01232 491731
Fax:	01232 642279

Combining features of regional and national postgraduate councils, it is the Northern Ireland equivalent of the Welsh and Scottish Councils.

RCGP (Royal College of General Practitioners)

Address:	14 Princes Gate London SW7 1PU
Tel:	0171 581 3232
Fax:	0171 581 3047
e-mail	*info@rcgp.org.uk*

Website: *http://www.rcgp.org.uk*

Aims: to encourage, foster and maintain the highest possible standards in general medical practice.

Membership: by examination (MRCGP). There are plans for membership by assessment of performance. It is organized on a faculty structure in the UK. There are overseas faculties.

Its Royal Charter entitles it to:

- establish and maintain an academic and education headquarters for GPs
- establish and maintain regional faculties and other organizations to further its objectives
- encourage persons of ability to enter medicine and become GPs
- undertake/assist with training courses and educational activities to enhance the medical knowledge and skill of GPs
- grant postgraduate diplomas or other certificates, establish chairs and lectureships, award prizes
- encourage publication of GP research and undertake/facilitate research
- diffuse information and hold meetings/courses on all GP matters
- co-operate with other interested bodies.

Publications include the *British Journal of General Practice* (monthly), an excellent and wide-ranging series of occasional papers and reports from general practice, educational packs, information sheets on a wide range of health and NHS issues and books. A publication list is obtainable from the Publications Department of the College.

The Information Service of the College provides library and information facilities to members, public representatives and voluntary groups related to primary care as well as maintaining a museum and archive.

SCOPME (Standing Committee on Postgraduate Medical Education)

Contact: Dr Jolyon Oxley (Secretary)
                  1 Park Square West
                  London NW1 4LJ

Tel: 0171 935 3916

Fax: 0171 935 8601

e-mail: *j.oxley@scopme.org.uk*

SCOPME was established by the Secretary of State for Health in August 1988 to replace the Council for Postgraduate Medical Education in England and Wales. It advises the Secretary of State on the delivery of postgraduate medical and dental education, taking into account the standards promulgated by professional bodies and the potential difficulties of reconciling service and training needs; it also identifies particular problems, and develops realistic solutions to these in consultation with relevant interests, and reports regularly. Its remit is for England only. Members are appointed by the Secretary of State, not as representatives of their respective disciplines. It meets five times per year. Working groups co-opt other experts to assist.

In addition to its informative annual reports it has conducted workshops, convened working parties, published reports and compiled recommendations on:

- NHS expenditure on postgraduate education
- study leave resourcing and uptake
- the needs of junior hospital doctors
- appraisal
- the content, management and monitoring of postgraduate education
- the educational implications of government health policy
- teaching doctors to teach
- multiprofessional education.

Scottish Council for Postgraduate Medical and Dental Education

Contact: Dr Graham Buckley (Executive Director)
                12 Queen Street
                Edinburgh EH2 1JE

Tel: 0131 225 4365

Fax: 0131 225 5891

e-mail: *hq.scpmde@dial.pipex.com*

The Council was established in 1970 by the Secretary of State for Scotland to:

- advise him
- provide a forum for discussion and co-ordination of arrangements for postgraduate medical and dental education in Scotland
- review and foster progress in vocational and continuing education for doctors and dentists in Scotland and to consider criteria for approval of training posts
- liaise with the (five) regional committees.

It was reconstituted in 1993 as a special health board which enabled it to take on executive responsibilities. In particular, the Scottish Council now holds the budget for the salaries and study leave for all doctors and dentists training in Scotland.

SIMG (Societas Internationalis Medicinae Generalis – The International Society of General Practice)

Founded in Vienna in 1959 by an Austrian GP, it amalgamated with WONCA Europe in 1995 to form the European Society of General Practice/Family Medicine.

SLOVTS (South London Organization of Vocational Training Schemes)

Contact:	Mrs Carlisle (Education Coordinator)
	Room 10
	Gassiot House
	St Thomas' Hospital
	London SE1 7EH
Tel:	0171 922 8250
Fax:	0171 922 8257
e-mail:	*j.chant@umds.ac.uk*

A joint organization set up to improve, expand and integrate vocational training in South London, combining the schemes based on Guys and St Thomas', Lewisham and King's. Aims to attract young GPs to stay in the city.

UKRA (UK Conference of Regional Advisers in General Practice)

Contact:	UKRA Secretary
	c/o RCGP
	14 Princes Gate
	London SW7 1PU
Tel:	0171 581 3232
Fax:	0171 581 3047
e-mail:	*pwlane@sheffield.ac.uk*
Membership:	Regional Directors and Associates and representatives of the ACO, NAGPT, GMSC, RCGP and other interests.

To provide a broadly based forum for the development of innovative approaches to postgraduate education for general practice.

UEMO (Union Européen des Médicins Omni-Practiciens)

Represents the interests of general practitioners within the EC structures. It may be contacted through EURACT, BMA or RCGP.

The Welsh Council for Postgraduate Medical and Dental Education

Contact: Dr Simon Smail (Sub-Dean for General Practice)
                  University of Wales College of Medicine
                  Department of Postgraduate Studies
                  Heath Park
                  Cardiff CF4 4XN

Tel: 01222 743087

Fax: 01222 754996

It was established by the Secretary of State for Wales, to advise him and to make provision for the delivery of postgraduate and continuing medical and dental education in Wales. There are four standing committees including the General Practice Standing Committee.

WONCA (World Organization of National Colleges, Academies and Academic Associations of General Practitioners/Family Physicians)

Contact: WONCA Secretariat
                  Locked Bag 11
                  Collins Street East Post Office
                  Melbourne, Victoria 8003
                  Australia

Tel: 61003 9650 0235

Also known as the World Organization of Family Doctors, it is a non-governmental organization with official relations with WHO and UNICEF. It was founded in Melbourne in 1972 as a result of a world conference.

Aims: to improve the quality of life of the peoples of the world through fostering and maintaining high standards of care in general practice/family medicine. It holds an international conference every three years. There are four standing committees, on medical education and audit, research, classification of primary care problems, and practice management.

Publications: *International classification of health problems in primary care* (OUP); *International classification of process in primary care* (OUP); FAMLI, a database of literature in primary care journals not listed in *Index Medicus* (College of Family Physicians, Canada); *The assessment of competence in general family practice* (MTP); *WONCA news* (OUP) – a supplement to *Family Practice*.

Sample regional policy for vocational training (Mersey Region)

The following subsection is reproduced by kind permission of Dr A Mathie, Regional Adviser, Mersey Region.

Overall aims for vocational training for general practice in the Mersey Region.

1 To produce competent, caring doctors able to function effectively in the system of primary care that is developing in the UK.
2 To produce doctors who are competent in, and motivated towards, continuous self-directed learning and development in their professional life.

Course organizers: core values and beliefs

1 Training promotes and enhances the belief that general practice is:
   - a complex and distinct medical specialty, integrating and encompassing appropriate parts of other disciplines
   - a fundamental activity set within the wider medical scene
   - centred on the patient and respects his/her autonomy and encompasses the traditional role of the healer within society.
2 The learner is pre-eminent, leading to training that:
   - promotes personal development and self-directed learning
   - satisfies the learner's needs and is learner driven
   - promotes problem-solving skills and critical reasoning
   - gives sensitive feedback on progress
   - gives a broad, near-reality, experience
   - provides a good model for practice.
3 Education emphasizes process and skills as much as content.
4 Course organizers respect trainees as professional colleagues.
5 General practice can only be truly learned in a general practice setting.
6 Specifically training doctors for general practice is beneficial for patient care.
7 Specific vocational training also helps doctors cope realistically with the demands and pressures of general practice.
8 Well-trained GPs will use finite resources effectively and monitor their own performance.

Mission statements

In the context of the trainee residential weekend and the trainee workshop, course organizers of Mersey Region will provide good-quality training and education for doctors who wish to consider a career in general practice and also those undergoing general professional training.

Course organizers of Mersey Region will provide good-quality training opportunities and courses for both potential and established trainers.

Responsibilities of course organizers

Course organizers recognize that they hold responsibility for only one strand of the training of future GPs. They acknowledge the pre-eminent influence of the training practice and the trainer in the development of trainees and the considerable contribution of the hospital training posts.

In considering responsibility for the trainee in the half-day release setting, course organizers see that they have a role that is educational, working within the constricting bounds of training, encouraging the developments of attributes and skills such as critical reasoning and analysis, problem solving, educational self-development, exploration and reflection. They also provide the potentially powerful learning experience of a small peer group. Within this setting trainees will be provided with opportunities to make adjustment from hospital to general practice medicine and to examine their preparedness for principalship. This opportunity is dependent upon the work experience of the trainee in his/her training practice.

Course organizers acknowledge that trainers hold the prime responsibility for the core content of trainee learning and also for both formative and summative assessment of individual trainees. They do, however, carry a responsibility for assessing the effectiveness of the workshops and their own personal performance.

The course organizer group has a responsibility to advise the regional adviser and the regional GP education committee on educational matters.

Course organizers have taken on further responsibilities in providing other courses for trainees, courses for trainers and potential trainers and the supervision of vocational training schemes.

Course organizers take an important role in trainer selection by offering informal advice to practices and contributing to formal visits to trainers and their practices.

Objectives for the trainees' half-day workshops

The trainee workshops will serve two main functions.

1 Adjustment. The workshop will help the process of transition from hospital to GP-based medicine. This is likely to involve attitudinal shifts that are unexpected and sometimes uncomfortable. This process is likely to be pre-eminent in the first six months of training.

2 Preparation. The workshop will help trainees prepare for the role of a principal in general practice by concentrating on problems generated from work and from perceived needs. The development of key skills will be encouraged such as consultation skills, critical self-audit etc.

In seeking to attain the above objectives, course organizers will concentrate mainly on the process of learning and develop their own skills in the fields of facilitation, setting climate, offering feedback and co-learning.

Books which course organizers have found useful

Course organizer colleagues around the UK and Ireland have recommended the following:

Active learning – a teacher's guide (1988) By J Baldwin and H Williams. Blackwell, Oxford. (Superb, well written.)

Adolescent health: training GP registrars (1996) By A McPherson, A McFarland and C Donovan. RCGP, London. (Authors include a veteran course organizer.)

Communicating with the public: a guide to those on the front line (1997) By M Kindred and M Goldsmith. (From the same stable as *Once upon a group ...*)

Developing assertiveness (1991) By A Townsend. Routledge, London. (It works, according to one course organizer's wife!)

Developing primary care: the academic contribution (1996) RCGP, London. (Don't be put off by the title – full of good stuff.)

Developing skills with people (1988) By S Dainow and C Bailey. John Wiley, Chichester. (Excellent ideas for courses on skills development.)

Doctor's communication handbook (2nd edn) (1997) By P Tate. Radcliffe Medical Press, Oxford.

Efficient care in general practice (1991) By GN Masch. Oxford University Press, Oxford. (Thought-provoking and challenging.)

Evidence-based general practice: a critical reader (1995) By L Ridsdale. Saunders, London.

53 interesting ways to appraise your teaching (1988) By G Gibbs *et al*. Technical and Educational Services, Bristol.

Handbook for medical teachers (1987) By D Newble and R Cannon. MTP, Lancaster. (Clear and concise guide to many teaching methods.)

Handbook for teachers in universities and colleges. Revised edn (1991) By D Newble and R Cannon. Kogan Page, London. (A guide to improving methods. Good on practicalities and assessment.)

Helping the client (1990) By J Heron. Sage, London. (Previously known as *A six category intervention analysis*.)

How to do it. BMA, London. (A practical three-volume guide to a huge range of non-clinical activities which doctors might have to undertake.)

How to manage your time (1987) By J Adair. Talbot-Adair, Guildford. (Life enhancing.)

How to read a paper: the basics of evidence-based medicine (1997) By T Greenhalgh. BMJ, London.

Inner apprentice, The (1996) By R Neighbour. Petroc Press, Newbury. (Now an established classic.)

Inner consultation, The (1987) By R Neighbour. Kluwer Academic, Lancaster. (Ditto.)

Managing change in primary care (1991) Edited by M Pringle. Radcliffe Medical Press, Oxford.

Management teams (1981) By R Meredith Belbin. Heinemann, Oxford. (Real team theory.)

Medical administration for front-line doctors (1990) By CA Pearson. FSG 57, Whitechapel Road, London. (Written by a pioneer in GP training in developing countries but applicable anywhere.)

New kind of doctor, A (1987) By J Tudor Hart. Merlin, London. (A classic; essential reading.)

New model of teaching and training, A (1994) By G Squires. Published by Squires, 186 Victoria Avenue, Hull. (Common sense brought to bear on educational theory.)

Paradox of progress, The (1994) By J Willis. Radcliffe Medical Press, Oxford.

RCGP occasional papers. A series of more than 70 monographs on primary care themes. Among these are some of particular relevance to vocational training, notably:

Trainee projects (RCGP Occasional Paper 29).

Priority objectives for general practice vocational training (RCGP Occasional Paper 30).

Course organizers in general practice (RCGP Occasional Paper 34).

Rating scales for vocational training (RCGP Occasional Paper 40).

Towards a curriculum for general practice training (RCGP Occasional Paper 44).

Portfolio-based learning in general practice (RCGP Occasional Paper 63).

Significant event auditing (RCGP Occasional Paper 70).

RCGP reports from general practice (A series of 30 working party reports on primary care themes. Especially interesting are Nos. 18–22 on *Prevention*, No. 23, *What sort of doctor?* and No. 27, *The nature of general medical practice*).

Some lives: a GP's East End (1991) By D Widgery. Sinclair Stevenson, London. (May become a classic?)

Teaching interpersonal skills – a handbook of experiential learning for health professionals (1989) By P Burnard. Chapman and Hall, London.

Teaching and learning communication skills in medicine (1998) By S Kurtz, J Silverman and J Draper. Radcliffe Medical Press, Oxford.

Teamwork for primary and shared care: a practical handbook (1994) By P Pritchard. Oxford University Press, Oxford.

The uncertain physician: dilemmas and decisions in medical practice (1987) By K Link. McFarland & Co Inc, USA.

The Irish scene

The following are all available from the Irish College of General Practitioners in Dublin:

Aims and objectives for vocational training for general practice teachers (A guide for course directors, tutors and trainees.)

Guidelines and recommendations for VT schemes in Ireland (A guide for steering committees, trainees and hospital teachers.)

Guidelines and recommendations for trainers and their practices (A guide for steering committees, course directors and trainees.)

Journals of relevance to vocational training

Education for General Practice. Radcliffe Medical Press, Oxford. (Formerly the *Journal of the Association of Course Organizers*.) Articles heavy and light on all aspects of postgraduate education. Published quarterly by Radcliffe. Free to members of the Association of Course Organizers.

Education for Health: change in training and practice. Replaces *Annals of Community-oriented Education*. First issued in 1988 as the official journal of the Network of Community Oriented Educational Institutions for Health Sciences. Publisher: Carfax, Abingdon. Editorial address: Professor Charles Engel, Institute of Education, University of London, 55–59 Gordon Square, London WC1H 0NT.

European Journal of General Practice. For and about general practitioners in Europe, it is the journal that represents the European Society for General Practice/Family Medicine. They have made it easy for us by writing it all in English! Publisher: Mediselect Publishing. Editorial address: Mediselect Publishing, PO Box 28091, 3828 ZH Hoogland, Netherlands.

Journal of General Internal Medicine. The official journal of the Society of General Internal Medicine. Editorial address: Veterans Affairs Medical Center (JGIM-III), University and Woodlands Avenues, Philadelphia, PA 19104, USA.

Journal of Family Practice. The main journal of family medicine – one of two domains of primary care in the United States, the other being general internal medicine. Publisher: Appleton & Lang, Stamford, CA, USA. Editorial address: 1650 Pierce Street, Denver, CO 80214, USA.

Medical Education. The international journal of undergraduate, postgraduate and continuing medical education, affiliated to the World Federation for Medical Education. Publisher: Blackwell Science. Editorial address: AMEE, 484 Perth Road, Dundee DD2 1LR.

British Journal of General Practice. Formerly the journal of the RCGP and the first reputable journal of research and education by GPs for GPs and probably the world leader. Publisher: RCGP. Editorial address: RCGP (Editorial office), 14 Princes Gate, London SW7 1PU.

Medical Teacher. The official journal of AMEE (see above).

Minimum educational criteria for training practices (with implementation dates in brackets)

1 All medical records and hospital correspondence must be filed in practice notes in date order (January 1984).
2 Appropriate medical records must contain easily discernible drug therapy lists for patients on long-term therapy (January 1986).
3 • Deaneries should set and publish targets for the achievement of summaries in medical records in teaching practices
   • Practices should be seen to be making progress towards reaching these targets
   • Slow progress in an otherwise satisfactory practice should lead to a shorter duration of re-approval than the regional norm
   • Joint Committee visitors will expect to receive the deanery's policy statements on summaries in medical records and will review and report on progress in implementation of the policy (January 1987).
4 All training practices should be developing methods for monitoring prescribing habits as an important part of the audit process (January 1986).
5 All training practices should have a library containing a selection of books and journals relevant to general practice (January 1987).
6 All training practices must provide opportunities for trainees to become familiar with the principles of medical audit and to participate in medical audit; and they must be able to demonstrate that trainees have actually done so (April 1991).

262 • Educating the future GP

7 All training practices must provide access to and use video cameras with their trainees (January 1996).

8 Formative assessment, that is, assessment for educational purposes, should form an essential part of all posts approved or selected for general practitioner training (January 1993).

9 Deaneries will be expected to ensure that their trainers are well placed to facilitate the technical and administrative aspects of the implementation of summative assessment (May 1997).

Procedure for obtaining certification on completion of training

Before any candidate can perform the duties of a general practitioner in any capacity, he or she must acquire a Certificate of Prescribed or Equivalent Experience. The essential steps are as follows:

1 Form VTR2 is a statement of satisfactory completion of an approved hospital post. It is signed by the hospital consultant and one must be furnished in respect of each contributory post. A special VTR2 statement must be completed for any hospital post held in the Republic of Ireland.

2 Form VTR1 is a statement of satisfactory completion of an approved general practice training post. If more than one is undertaken separate VTR1 forms must be obtained, signed by the respective trainers.

'Satisfactory completion' is defined as 'completion of that period of training in such a manner as to have acquired the medical experience which may reasonably be expected to be acquired from training of that duration in that employment' (NHS (Vocational Training) Regulations 1997, 9(1)).

3 VTR1 and VTR2 forms should be sent to the Director of Postgraduate General Practice Education along with a copy of the annual GMC registration certificate.

4 The Regional Director may then issue a Certificate of Satisfactory Completion of Training. Evidence of passing Summative Assessment completes the documentation to be sent to the Joint Committee.

5 If the Joint Committee are satisfied that the applicant has acquired the prescribed experience, they shall issue the candidate a certificate of prescribed experience. If they are not satisfied they shall issue a statement setting out the reasons why they are not satisfied.

Experience gained abroad or outside the network of approved training posts may count towards vocational training. Application may be made through the Secretary of the Joint Committee for recognition of 'equivalent experience'.

The JCPT Certificate is the mandatory licence to undertake general practice in the NHS. Certified completion of vocational training may be registered with the General Medical Council on application to the Registration Division.

Guidelines on study leave for GP trainees

Vocational training in hospital posts

Professional or study leave is granted for postgraduate purposes approved by employing authorities and includes study (usually, not exclusively or necessarily on a course), research, teaching, examining or taking an examination, visiting clinics and attending professional conferences.

Study leave must normally be granted to the maximum extent consistent with maintaining services. Juniors should always ensure that their study leave applications are countersigned by their consultants, which in most cases should ensure that it is consistent with maintaining services.

The recommended periods of study leave for SHOs and registrars are either day release with pay and expenses for the equivalent of one day a week during the university term, or a maximum of 30 days a year with pay and expenses. Leave with pay and expenses (other than exam fees) for the purpose of sitting an exam for higher qualifications is granted in addition to the 30 days a year.

The half day included as part of a vocational training scheme does not use up all the 30 days. There should be approximately 15 days a year for study leave for other purposes.

Study leave does not have to be related to the SHO job that the trainee is doing at the time (this applies to DIY trainees too) but this is sometimes given as the reason why study leave is refused. If this happens you should appeal against the decision as it is not in the interests of trainees or of higher professional training for this to happen.

Expenses. When employing authorities grant study leave they must also grant pay and expenses; they cannot grant study leave without pay and expenses. In general, the full rates of travel and subsistence negotiated in the General Whitley Council should be paid. Where these rates are not paid in full, the authority concerned must not have a pre-determined policy of paying reduced expenses, such as paying only 50% of all travel claims; they must make a decision in response to an individual application.

Appeals. If study leave is refused, or granted without appropriate pay and/or expenses, junior doctors can take the following steps (BMA members are advised always to consult their regional offices):

- appeal to the Regional Study Leave Committee. This is a committee of the regional health authority, on which regional Hospital Junior Staff Committees are represented, whose job it is to ensure consistent and uniform practices and to hear and decide appeals. It should be noted that referral of refused applications is not automatic

- go to the Small Claims Court. One or two successful instances of this have been reported to the BMA. Small claims procedure was introduced in England and Wales to enable either party to a claim for less than £500 to have the case dealt with by arbitration. The hearings are usually in private and much less formal than court proceedings. A booklet giving details and called *Small Claims in the County Court* is available on request from any county court office
- employing authority appeals (only in cases where expenses have been stopped or reduced). Because employing authorities have some discretion in deciding what levels of expenses can be paid, the DHSS has in the past argued that employees may not appeal beyond employing authority level. Although the BMA does not accept this ruling, and is challenging it, it is often worth appealing to the employing authority in cases where pre-determined policies are being imposed in contravention of the above rules.

Vocational training in general practice

Study leave should be equivalent to that available to hospital SHOs. Each region has different study leave arrangements but in areas where there is a full day-release scheme this may result in registrars being refused other related study leave.

The trainer as the employer has the right to grant or refuse study leave and there is no right of appeal. It is advisable therefore to include study leave provisions in the contract between the trainer and trainee. The BMA trainee model contract has provision for 30 days' study leave during the trainee year.

Expenses. Registrars should continue to be paid normally for the time spent on study leave. Apart from course fees and travel to and from examinations, all expenses are reimbursed under section 63 arrangements. Course fees are paid automatically and examination fees come from a separate budget. Each region has a budget for section 63 expenditure which is cash limited for all GPs including trainees. Regions annually allocate a fixed sum from the budget for each doctor, the amount varies between regions. If, at the end of the financial year, there is money available because some doctors have not spent their allowance in full, this is used to reimburse those doctors who have claimed more than the allowance. It is important that all registrars claim their expenses as some budgets are underspent. Some regions have arranged for certain courses to have first call on the available resources and therefore for these reimbursement will be in full. You will be notified of the arrangements in your region by the regional director or your course organizer.

Travel to or from examinations is funded separately.

Appeal. A contractual agreement to allow a specific amount of study leave is legally binding, and it is therefore advisable for the trainee and trainer to sign a contract which identifies the study leave arrangements. Most disagreements occur where study leave has not been specified in a contract or no contract exists.

When problems do occur your course organizer and the regional director can usually help. If it is a persistent problem then they can bring pressure to bear which may result in the withdrawal of approval from the trainer. The registrar post is supernumerary and therefore absence on study leave should not affect the smooth running of the practice.

Source documents: *Terms and conditions of service for GPs*, paras 250–4; BMA (1994) *Junior doctors' handbook*. BMA, London; GMSC (1996) *Study leave for GP registrars*. GMSC, GP Registrars Subcommittee, BMA, London.

Data Protection Act (1984)

If you are using a computer system to process data about *living individuals*, from which an individual *can be identified* (e.g. name, address), then there is a legal obligation on you, the data user, to ensure that your computer system complies with the principles of the Data Protection Act (1984).

Briefly, the principles are as follows.

1 Personal data must be obtained and processed fairly and lawfully.
2 They must be held only for one or more specified and lawful purpose(s), i.e. in accordance with the data user's (compulsory) registration.
3 They must not be used or disclosed in any manner incompatible with the registered purpose(s).
4 The data must not be excessive in relation to the purpose(s) for which they are held.
5 Data must be accurate and, where necessary, kept up to date.
6 Data must not be kept for longer than necessary.
7 An individual is entitled to have access to any personal data relating to him/her, and if necessary to have such data corrected or erased.
8 Appropriate security measures must be taken by the data user against accidental or unauthorized access to, or alteration, disclosure or destruction of, personal data.

To ensure that your system complies with the principles you may require further details. Guidelines to the Act can be obtained free of charge from:

The Data Protection Registrar,
Springfield House,
Water Lane,
Wilmslow,
Cheshire SK9 5AX.

Other data users will be entitled to insist that systems with which they share data are registered under the Act.

Part 6

Training for general practice:
health for all?

Overview

The focus of this book has been on the needs of the course organizer and the group of trainees who make up the vocational training day-release course. It is now fashionable to talk about seamless medical education from student days to retirement. There is a spectrum of learning settings but the range of educators involved have much in common.

The final chapter asserts that the seamless garment is much more extensive than our everyday experience would suggest. Just as institutional boundaries introduce spurious divisions between the various sets of teachers of general practice, we feel separated from our counterparts in other parts of the world by the artefacts of differing national systems. Transcending these boundaries is liberating and shows us that sharpening our focus and narrowing our field of view sacrifices perspective. As educators and clinicians we all operate in an interdependent, changing world. There is a heightened sense of this at the turn of one millennium to another.

Finally, Meeke and Best attempt to review their journey to date and look beyond.

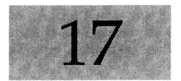

General practice training:
the wider context

'No man is an island, entire of itself; every man is a piece of the Continent, a part of the main...' (John Donne, Meditation XVII)

The all-encompassing, all-providing NHS has kept the eyes of GPs in the UK fixed firmly inwards. Few of our neighbouring countries have anything to compare with it, conceptually, at least.

There has been a decade of continuing change in the NHS. For GPs this shows no sign of coming to an end and has absorbed much of our energies. Not surprisingly the perspective of GP teachers is dominated by the changing training agenda inherent in NHS practice. It is not unnatural that island-dwellers should tend to be insular, it is simply not necessary. There must be other reasons for this perspective. After all, the means of international communication have never been more accessible, yet to the bulk of our trainees the world of primary care outside these shores is a closed book. There are signs that this is changing. The recruitment crisis of the 1990s in the UK has revealed two trends:

1 the influx of young continental graduates seeking training here, filling up vacant places and, indeed, rescuing a proportion of our schemes from oblivion
2 the numbers of trainees who decline the path of their predecessors – that of going into lifelong partnerships at the first opportunity. Increasing numbers are electing to seek experience elsewhere for a time before committing themselves to what seems like the life-sentence of the GP contract.

The evidence-based and critical reading emphasis in recent years has alerted trainees to the existence of a world literature of primary health care issues. The epidemiological perspective is opening our minds. Other influences from far-off places impinge on our consciousness increasingly – the AIDS pandemic and the recent impact of food-borne disease, for example animal pathogens and the prion, must alert us to the global issues of medical environmentalism. The threat of multiple resistant tuberculosis is directly related to the aspects of health care systems in the USA and the Third World. What are the consequences for our approach to infectious disease when 25% of our population annually visit countries where antibiotics may be obtained without prescription or restriction?

General practice differs greatly from other medical specialties in its tendency to insularity. Historically, the international impact of our medical culture has been based on two institutional concepts – the hospital and the laboratory. Both are European inventions which spread through the dominance of Europe in international politics and trade from the 16th to the 19th century.

Congruent institutional structures and modes of thinking therefore emerged in all continents, marginalizing the immense diversity of indigenous treatment cultures which exist everywhere and relegating them to the status of folk medicine. Health care in Africa and Asia was until recently based on doctor-led hospitals which would be recognizable by doctors from medical schools everywhere.

The barriers to medical internationalism were not institutional but linguistic. Lines of communication were based on language blocks and migration patterns, not proximity. Thus, the British pattern was carried with the far-flung empire; likewise the French. The Germanic medical culture followed the Teutonic diaspora throughout Eastern Europe, greatly influencing the Russian Empire. The burgeoning population of North America assimilated, through migration, influences from all three. This resulted in a variety of medical cultures which, nevertheless, had a common institutional core.

The hospital and the laboratory converge in the medical school. This produced a more or less universal consensus about what constituted the formation and training of the generic doctor. Archetypical medical school products were in a position to staff the hospital-centred systems of the world, interchangeable apart from language barriers. This cohesion has been breaking down in the latter half of the 20th century. Discernible influences include:

- the recent assertion of alternative medical culture – folk medicine is undergoing a renaissance as local ethnic identities become more assertive. People are becoming disillusioned with the power and rigidity of conventional medicine, regarded by many as 'colonial', and are turning to 'alternative medicine'
- Western medicine has performed poorly in the Third World through reliance on the hospital and disease-centred perspectives. Unprecedented levels of poverty, famine and social disintegration, ascribable to the international economic order, are a destabilizing force in global politics
- the fragmentation of the 'Soviet Bloc' has resulted in economic upheavals in Eastern Europe and Asia, resulting in poverty, political instability and warfare with health consequences for the Eurasian landmass
- the collapse of the 19th century empires has led to the emergence of new alliances based on proximity rather than language – the European Union, the dollar zone, the 'Asian tiger' economies.

International structures have emerged, notably the World Health Organization, which seek to achieve an overview of health issues on a global scale. The declaration of Alma Ata, condensed to the soundbite 'Health for all by the year 2000', has resounded round the world. Unrealistic and utopian as it might be, it established a new agenda for medicine – to broaden the base of the health care pyramid and not just to build a higher one.

The triumphalism of medical science, dependent on high technology and heavy investment, is challenged by the need to deliver basic health care to whole populations. The triple strands of primary care – national health policy, public health medicine and community-based care – have been mandated to carry health out of the institutional setting and into every home.

We are part of this movement. As GPs, and especially as teachers of community-based medicine, we are in the forefront of this justice campaign. It lends enhanced meaning to what we do and may spark a sense of mission if we grasp the full context and its historic significance.

Low morale is well documented as the main threat to general practice in the UK as we approach the millennium. It is impinging on the quality of our health service (the recruitment crisis) and the attitudes of our trainees towards their career prospects ('voting with their feet'). In every part of the world the GP is seen as the second rank doctor and the growing discipline is hampered by under-resourcing, a poverty of appropriate research and development, and policies which seldom get beyond the stage of the consultative document or mission statement.

We, in these islands, are in a privileged position. Most countries in Europe and the developed world have never reformed their systems of primary care and still practise in the manner of the UK in the 1930s. There is a vicious circle of low social esteem, poor education, poor earnings and heavy competition (Boerma et al., 1993). The happy accident of the post-war health service has placed us in the forefront of primary care thought and potential. An introspective stance is a denial of this richness. We easily fail to appreciate its worth and we deny the prophetic power of the prayer 'health for all'.

This is not an evangelical call to spread the UK model of health care throughout the world. That would be to fall into the trap, once again, of colonial attitudes. The educational perspective should transcend cultural barriers – the disparity of health care systems, of language and economic interests, and this is where GP teachers have a unique contribution to make.

There are formidable obstacles to working in other countries as a GP. We now have the right of mobility throughout Europe, but soon encounter the barrier of language. General practice, though universal in its concepts, is heavily dependent on the continuity and intimacy of the personal consultation. A scientist may be able to function quickly and adequately in a foreign laboratory, but a GP has little hope of conducting an adequate consultation in an unfamiliar cultural and linguistic setting.

Even in countries which have obvious affinities in their respective cultures there are barriers. For example, there is substantial divergence between the UK and USA because of the wide disparity of view about the nature and organization of health care – as a commodity or right of citizenship, based on access to specialists (ambulatory medicine) or the GP (family medicine). Everywhere the GP is intimately related to the welfare and social security infrastructure of the society. These barriers are more substantial in primary care than in the institutional setting of the laboratory, hospital or medical school. Therefore we are not training GPs for export like the medical missionaries of old. What, then, is this unique contribution of the GP teacher?

It can be seen as operating at three levels:

1 the liberal education of our trainees
2 the development of the specific discipline of education and training for primary care
3 outreach to assist in the tasks of training family doctors in other societies and systems.

The liberal education of the learner

The liberal education of the learner is a curriculum issue. Increasing forces conspire to narrow our perspective to the practicalities of the present – the here and now issues as defined by government policy and examination syllabus. Life can be injected into these by appreciation of the wider context.

Example I: Medical economics

This is an important curriculum feature in preparation for the primary care-led NHS. It can be dealt with through teaching about the theory of management, financial administration and regulatory framework, areas which most person-centred clinicians wish to avoid. In any case, like fundholding, they are subject to transition, fashion and change.

Alternatively, the universalities of medical economics could be the focus – a more enduring set of concepts which might be applied to this, or the next, major challenge. This would entail consideration of the ethical questions of health rationing, the gate-keeper versus patient advocate role of the GP, prioritizing the use of health resources and manpower with analysis of health care paradigms drawn from other major systems – discerning the values enshrined differentially in each. This might lead to the development of a simple summative construct such as 'medical economics in a nutshell', as formulated and stated by a local GP at a course in Derry.

'Health care systems should represent three qualities – they should be good, handy and cheap.' Applying this aphorism to what we do is a useful stimulus for discussion when applied to our own system and compared with others.

- The UK system is good and cheap, but not handy (problem – access to secondary care; rationing through waiting lists).
- The US system is good and handy but not cheap (so it is most productive for those with money and good health).
- The Soviet system was quite good, handy and cheap but only because it did not pay its doctors and nurses well and, in a free market, it is collapsing.

These values can then be applied to the microcosm of the locality commissioner or the trainee GP as a learning exercise. How do you tackle the problems of waiting lists locally? How do you improve patient access at the surgery when your appointment system is under pressure? How do you improve quality of acute care when there is no extra money available and your practice team is saturated with health promotion activities?

Example II: Appropriate technology

Our dominant medical culture is disease centred and appreciative of technological progress. This served us well during times of economic growth. Now all of the technologically advanced societies are discovering that their economies cannot put into practice the techniques which science has produced – we cannot afford the population-wide implications of our capability. This is a painful discovery especially when it is compounded by the by-products of the technology. These problems are no longer remote from GPs. High-tech embryology has faced every GP with questions about the management of infertility. The considerable cost of controlling fertility is being overshadowed by the cost of producing individual pregnancies, not to mention the spin-off problems surrounding how genetic material is treated.

For the first time we are looking to lessons learned in the Third World generations ago (King, 1966) such as:

- when you cannot afford health care what you do is health education
- when you have more patients than doctors can treat you allow nurses (and health auxiliaries) to exercise greater responsibilities
- when the chips are down, restrictive practices have to go – it is more important to fight disease than argue about who does what
- when the lights go out we are all in the dark – complex machines are dependent on expensive infrastructure and are therefore vulnerable
- institutional-based medicine does not solve the health problems of the community – it serves well those who have access to the institution
- those with expensive, long, complex training are wasted in the front line – they should be problem-solvers, backing up and facilitating a rank of less differentiated workers
- if you have a choice between an expensive remedy and a cheap one, why use the expensive one?

- people have responsibility for their own health. The state has responsibilities, but limited resources and difficult choices
- health care provision is not primarily a business.

One can recognize how the need for change is forcing us to incorporate these ideas into our education and practice. The monolithic disease-centred undergraduate curriculum is crumbling. It is being revised to emphasize epidemiology rather than pathology, problem-based rather than subject-based learning, and training in the community rather than 'centres of excellence'.

Vocational training is more than ever focused on health promotion, prevention and actions guided by evidence of efficacy and cost effectiveness. Public policy is embracing the concept of bottom-up rather than top-down priority setting. The priorities in allocation of resources should be based on making the community diagnosis (locality commissioning) rather than letting specialists display their wares for community consumption.

In summary, the appropriate (or intermediate) technology perspective holds that higher technology is expensive, dependent on complex infrastructural support, requires high-level skills to operate and maintain, is brittle, usually dependent on distant suppliers and creates centralization. Lower technology is inexpensive, requires less infrastructure, fewer skills to operate and maintain, is home produced and more likely to be widely dispersed. The decision to use high tech should therefore be deliberate and based on defensible reasoning. Otherwise low tech is better.

For example, high-tech capability fuels expensive expectations which contribute towards expensive litigation – 'The plaintiff had headaches yet you did not order a brainscan, Doctor'. The high-tech imperative is largely responsible for the closure of neighbourhood hospitals.

Adopting the intermediate technology emphasis influences our choices at every level of practice:

- planning premises with multi-use space
- team work employing nurse practitioners and health ancillaries
- prescribing practices.

It may be as important to our educational approach as is evidence-based practice. The limitations of low technology are evident. Those of high technology become obvious when something goes wrong. This perspective has much in common with the 'green' environmentalist stance.

Developing primary care training

One thing teachers of general practice need is perspective. Most of the chapters of this book have implicitly addressed the problem of 'not being able to see the wood for the trees' – how to reduce the boundless discipline of general practice to a manageable set of prioritized tasks and work out a division of labour between the course organizer, trainer and hospital.

Defining the boundaries is a demanding task. Paradoxically, this is facilitated by rejecting the restriction of thought imposed by boundaries in order to explore the unknown. Unfortunately course organizers do not have access to a generous travel budget and there is little available guidance for the journey.

Fortunately, much of the exploring can be done by your fireside with journals or on the Net. A few generalities will become clear.

1 A characteristic of general practice is that it is heavily influenced by the health care system and culture of the country. This contrasts with hospital or laboratory medicine for the reasons outlined earlier. It is only through scrutinizing the systems that operate elsewhere that one can achieve a critical appraisal of the system operating in one's own country (Buckley and Heyrmann, 1994). Reflecting on the differences can be a great antidote for low morale. It may also generate ideas which inform your approach to training for the changing times in the UK.

2 However various the role of the GP is in different jurisdictions it is clear that there is a large core of activities that are carried out everywhere. When you observe a consultation, even in a foreign language, you will find little need for an interpreter to know what is going on.

3 This core of general practice activity represents the essence of primary care. Any variation in this represents different emphases which are subject to local influences and factors.

4 The tasks of the educators for primary care in different jurisdictions are strikingly similar. It is astonishing to find that whilst, as a GP, you may not be talking the same language, as teachers there is instant rapport and empathy.

5 Discussing your challenges as a teacher with a foreigner forces you to define closely what you do and mean. This is a reflective process which enables you to make discoveries. For example, discussing the nature of your curriculum with a North American immediately reveals the strengths and weaknesses of relying on structured learning objectives. Explaining to an Eastern European how we train for person-centred practice is equally revealing of how you define your terms, processes and aims. Most training systems do not have a course organizer. It can be a humbling experience to explain why one is necessary here!

6 As with evolution there are reasons behind all apparent differences in systems – they have each adapted to their own environment. The reflection on differences reveals positive lessons. For example, many Eastern European GPs have a highly developed interest in occupational health because the former regimes emphasized the need to service the industrial workforce. This perspective is poorly reflected here, where the factory doctor tends to be a GP employed part-time to police absenteeism. Many doctors in the Third World are very skilled in health education techniques because part of their job is to train and support village health workers.

7 The same task can be done in different ways. We tend to teach consultation and communication, minor surgery and CPR skills in isolation from one another. In the Netherlands there are highly developed multi-media skills laboratories servicing the problem-based learning curriculum for students. Trainees can get access to these and learn at their own pace through recurrent visits to the skill laboratory.

8 Promotion of research and development flourishes on the diet of questions raised by comparing how things are done in different systems and settings.

9 Course organizing skills are honed by the comparative process of meeting a foreign peer. It is an exercise in mutual learning/teaching between equals in active listening, in defining and clarifying and in non-evaluative criticism. When you fall into a points scoring exercise it is time to go home – you have ceased being a learner.

10 If you venture into this kind of situation abroad as a GP educator you are contributing to the development of training here, since all the benefits are likely to be mutual. Be warned – you are liable to be asked to give a little talk to the faculty/trainee group/local CME meeting while you are here. Globe-trotting teachers 'sing for their supper', and learn a few songs in order to do so. Development of your own discipline and personal skills are a useful product of such outreach.

'Europe is a patch-work of contrasting cultures and health care systems.' (Sips, 1995)

Outreach development

There are increasing opportunities for undertaking the broadening of your horizons, career and skills development and at the same time contributing to the development of primary care training in foreign countries. There is a well-trodden path to North America and Australia/New Zealand to contribute to, or attend, conferences on primary care training, or to spend extended study leave in an academic department. Many countries in the Middle East have had primary care development programmes based in university departments. Accounts of these have featured in issues of *Education for General Practice*. There is a variety of sources of funding including the annual fellowship scheme of the ACO. The regional director and overseas department of the RCGP may be able to give advice on further opportunities.

The emphasis on primary health care development has been gathering pace with the declaration of Alma Ata and the WHO Charter for General Practice in Europe. Countries worldwide have realized that reliance on an excess of hospital facilities is less productive of health care than better resourced primary care. This has been seen with startling clarity with the collapse of the Soviet Bloc. A dozen or more 'new' republics appeared on the Eastern borders of the EU, all with aspirations to enter the union. This requires harmonization of economic and social organization and the attainment of performance indices. There was an avalanche of appeals to the EU headquarters in Brussels for financial and technical assistance to bring about reform of the old Soviet health care system which had been uniformly imposed throughout the former Eastern Bloc. This system was based on specialists and semi-specialists, mostly working from hospitals and their satellite polyclinics. It was characterized by overmanning, poor conditions of service and rigid restrictive practices.

Technical assistance programmes were rapidly put together. The main areas of activity were health management, health care finance, undergraduate medical education and primary care training. The skills and educational credentials of course organizers make them uniquely valuable to such programmes. The issues, challenges, background and approaches are clearly described by Lember (1996) and Kinworth (1994). These programmes provide fascinating case studies of the management of educational change and the application of crisis theory. The opportunity and need for change are evident, but mostly to the economic planners. The risks involved are keenly appreciated by the politicians, many of whom have an insecure hold on the reins of power. The costs of change are feared by health care professionals – the specialist/ hospital sector faces downsizing. Those in general (community-based) practice fear a tunnel of insecurity but are excited at the glimpse of light at the end. The population have only a tenuous appreciation of what all this signifies. The universities overproduce medical graduates most of whom are faced with unemployment. Their curriculum is rigidly based on bio-medical and clinical sciences. The educational priorities are clear-cut but formidable:

- to achieve the introduction of community-orientated medicine as the first step in reform of the university curriculum
- to establish a curriculum plan for training in family medicine
- to create a parallel training scheme for established practitioners who may never have had general medical training (specialization began during medical school in the old system, e.g. paediatricians followed a separate course from the second year onwards)
- to train GP teachers who will provide undergraduate and trainee attachments
- to advice the Ministry of Health on the implications of these changes in terms of regulation, eventual EU harmonization and resource allocation
- to advise the health insurance organization of the funding implications of establishing and sustaining postgraduate training and CME.

Frequently, these advisory functions are contracted out to different technical advice agencies (by competitive tendering through the EU in most cases). Co-ordinated progress is difficult to achieve. This depends heavily on the commitment to change and the capability of the Ministry of Health. Daunting as these tasks are, they challenge the course organizer to work from first principles and stark priorities to create three curricula.

1 Training the trainers in the skills of education and running a training practice.
2 Establishing a programme for trainees.
3 Creating a programme for retraining existing practitioners.

A major challenge is to focus on these tasks and not be deflected into trying to solve all the practical problems of wholesale health care reform for the whole country – a new perspective on respecting the autonomy of the learners, i.e. everyone concerned.

Other geographical zones present specific problems but none can be more challenging and interesting than Eastern Europe. For those who wish to rise to the challenge the following notes on three major geographical development zones are offered.

Notes on Third World countries: Africa

They tend to resent their status as Third World countries and are unsure what the term means except that they are at the bottom of the world economic heap. Often artificially determined by European colonial boundaries that have little meaning, their sense of nationhood is important but mostly in the sense of having removed the colonial structure and taking responsibility for their own future. Local 'tribal' identities have precedence over national identity. This is reflected in government where power struggles are between ethnic sub-groups rather than on ideological grounds. This gives rise to problems in decisions about resource allocation or redistribution. Mainly traditional, rural cultures, the grafting on of urban structures, institutional values and Western technology cause stresses which lead to malfunction of systems. The views of kinship, citizenship and property rights are rooted in rural, homogeneous sub-units. This leads to ethical values that are easily misunderstood by outsiders, compounded by the stark rich–poor divide.

The overwhelming reality is economic dependency – the inability to influence market forces, aspirations towards Westernized lifestyles and the reliance on imported technology. Gross national products are incapable of providing acceptable standards of education and health for all. They do have lively informal economies, considerable social stability outside the urban slums and functioning subsistence economy patterns in rural areas.

Conventional health care is a cash commodity. Government hospitals are urban, free and grossly overloaded. 'Mission in hospitals' are foreign benevolent institutions, mostly rural with satellite community health centres and, of necessity, charge fees for treatment. There is a separate system of medicine practised at community level based on religious belief systems and herbalism. It does not interact with the formal health structures but is more influential in determining health-seeking behaviour.

Progressive health policies are widely practised by government under severe limitations. Priorities are basic sanitation, clean water, health education, maternal and child care and disease eradication programmes. The health economy has been devastated by AIDS and the resulting need for high-tech responses to life-saving imperatives.

Health care workers

Universities are few and increasingly community orientated. Major treatment centres make enormous demands on the health economy and it is difficult to balance the health priorities. Doctors are attracted to private practice in urban areas or to emigration. Most health care is delivered by non-graduate health auxiliaries (medical assistants) and various kinds of nurses at village level. Junior doctors are drafted into district hospitals to keep the service going and few stay in public service.

The foreign aid agencies play a vital part in research, advice and community development for health. Increasingly, they are moving towards short-termism in the form of disaster relief and programmes with limited but visible outcomes that will look good back home.

Education issues

- Input to medical and paramedical training programmes.
- Respecting the indigenous attempts to grasp major problems in health care planning and facilitating appropriate training using appropriate technology.
- Influencing the medical ethos towards community congruence.
- Importing skills in management, administration, planning and appropriate intervention.
- Education for health, family autonomy, mutual assistance and community development.
- Training the trainers.

Notes on the Middle East

Countries vary greatly in size but are, on the whole, affluent. Government style tends to be patriarchal but concerned for health care development along European/American lines with 'centres of excellence' based on high technology, prestige hospitals and medical schools. These latter draw students from wide areas of the Islamic world.

Islamic tradition demands respect and penalties for breaches of norms can be severe especially in relation to gender issues and alcohol use. The common language among health care professionals is English. Community-based health care is growing rapidly through district hospital and satellite health centres and rural health programmes.

Medical training is increasingly open to women but they are still few. Mostly, they enter GP training where they outnumber men. Many trainees are seconded from the armed forces. The training process is based largely on supervised hospital/community clinical experience, and an academic block of study with an emphasis on public health medicine and a dissertation.

They have a unique advantage – the opportunity to create primary health care training programmes *de novo* and with expert expatriate advice rather than through internal reform of existing institutions.

Notes on Eastern Europe

Eastern Europe is not the Third World, as they have been technologically advanced societies with a tradition of medicine which has the same roots as the rest of Europe. Their aspirations are similar. They are experiencing responsibility for their own health care system for the first time in three generations and are reacting to their former experience of the centralized command economy. Their existing system works because of the skills and dedication of health care professionals despite very low pay and difficult conditions.

In general, the status of doctors is low and their income less than average. Their self-esteem is rooted in pride in what they do and this is often related to specialist status. Restrictive practices are widespread due to overproduction of doctors and there is a weak understanding of the nature of general practice/family medicine. It is not professionally respected and it is under-represented in the curriculum of the medical schools. Social medicine is established as clinical epidemiology with a university perspective.

Specialists also practise in the community – outreach from the hospital via the polyclinic. The medical organizations are specialist dominated and the GPs, who share the polyclinic with the specialists, are seen as referral agents. Many of these are physicians who failed to achieve higher level specialist examinations. The functions of a GP are divided between generalist paediatrician, generalist gynaecologist and generalist physician and some function in industrial settings. They do not have control over their premises, there is no primary care team and social services are patchy. Nurses function mainly as receptionists and are paid out of the GP's income. Nursing skills are under-developed. Medical schools are hierarchical and conservative. The curriculum is focused on the medical sciences, clinical experience for medical students is limited and hospital based and GPs are not paid for teaching attachments. Teaching is not a right or duty of a doctor – it has been strictly regulated under Communism and teachers have to be ratified by university or government officials.

Vocational training which consists of hospital experience, formal examinations and dissertations is in need of reform. There is no financial or administrative framework for practice-based training or payment for trainees and new social/medical insurance systems are multiple, under-funded and service centred. They may not budget for training. The priorities are:

- for the Ministry of Health
  - legislation on policy for health priorities
  - policy for training of generalists
- for health insurance companies, a budget for training
- for medical organizations, the need to recognize specialism of primary health care
- for universities, the need to reflect community perspectives and needs
- for GPs, the need to retrain:

Physician
Paediatrician } To become generalist primary physicians
Gynaecologist

Problems

Under-resourced
The process of retraining
Incentives to retrain
Medical unemployment
Generally proven systems for retraining slow to evolve

- the need to train new generalists from recent graduates

Problems

Poorly formed concept of general practice
Recruitment and difficulty in placing finished trainers in practices
Lack of training practices

- Specialists
  - excessive numbers; threat of redundancy
  - excess hospital capacity; closure of units
  - threatened by rise of a new specialty competing with them for polyclinic space
  - reduced referrals
  - specialist power blocks in university; examination system; and medical organizations.

Opportunities

- Good quality of medical graduates.
- Interest in Balint method opens the way to person-centred approaches.
- Need to shift resources from secondary to primary care for economic reasons.
- Need a gate-keeper function.

- Aspire to EU membership – need harmonization of structures.
- Resources available through EU funded programmes.

Values

- Patient centredness – emphasis on rehabilitation and care for workers in industrial setting.
- Much emphasis on 'holistic' approach – physical therapies, allergy treatments, convalescence, sanitoria.

What the course organizer can do

A final plea on breaking down insularity. The most used form of international learning/teaching for GPs is distance learning via the written word (soon to come routinely through cyber-space). Perhaps the best form of self-development for course organizers in these islands is to buy a multimedia PC, hook up the modem to the Net and e-mail and start networking with each other and with journals such as our own *Education for General Practice*. Perhaps I will begin to take my own advice concerning Internet working.

- Take opportunities to visit and attend medical conferences in other countries.
- Read widely – there are international journals on primary care, medical education, academic medicine and interdisciplinary education.
- Look at articles which describe training in foreign countries – there are increasing numbers of these in our own journal (*Education for General Practice*). Recent ones include the Middle East, Baltic States, Russian Federation, New Zealand and Australia.
- Try to get an impression about the structure of health care in key countries, especially the EU territories (since we have open borders with them); would trainees benefit from knowing about this?
- Find out how GPs are trained in other territories.
- Join EURACT – an excellent way of identifying your own problems in training and comparing notes on how they are solved elsewhere.
- Compare and contrast.
- Bring visitors to your course and let the trainees 'pick their brains'.
- We live in a multicultural society and trainees need to be sensitized to transcultural issues.

It may be that no man is an island but quite a lot of course organizers feel isolated; there are more ways than one to break out.

Scenario: Ends and trends

Best: *So what did you think of the annual course organizers' conference?*

Meeke: *It was a lot of fun, but a bit confusing. Nobody seemed to be in the same situation as anybody else. Everybody has a different approach, and every region is different too. It took a while to see that the same few themes kept recurring – problems in running group work, integrating SHOs, knowing what the job description is, and how to keep all the plates spinning at the same time. Some people seemed to know all the in-words. I felt stupid having to get them all spelled out. I've come back with a notebook full of acronyms, definitions and a few good ideas. There was a lot of talk about stress – mostly worries about time, priorities and the impact of all that CO work on home life and leisure.*

Best: *It used to be unfashionable to admit to stress. Maybe that's what you should be looking at now that you have the prospect of some free time. What else have you learned? Did you get any impressions about where vocational training is going – what are the growth points?*

Meeke: *There seemed to be three kinds of people – those who were deep into group work, those who were into administration of training schemes and the rest of us who were struggling to break the surface of both.*

Best: *Yes, that's every year's story, but often there are signs of new directions.*

Meeke: *There was a lot of talk about redefining course organizers. Some expect that in a few years we'll be integrated with CME tutors, maybe as associate directors, bridging the divide between vocational training and continuing medical education. At the same time, many think there will be a convergence of regional postgraduate councils and universities in departments of postgraduate general practice with the new course organizers as honorary lecturers (or some such grade) so that there is a pooling of resources between undergraduate teachers, research academics, vocational training and continuing medical education teachers.*

Best: *What was the feeling about that?*

Meeke: *Split, I would say; some suspicion about the universities getting too much hold on professional education with their own agenda, mostly related to funding. Many were very enthusiastic about recognition of academic status and access to research facilities, but felt that the job brief of a generic GP educator would be too broad for comfort. A lot seem to be doing higher degrees, so they must feel that there is a developing career path in GP education.*

Best: *What about the jobbing course organizer. Is he going to be a thing of the past? I'd be concerned about that. It would introduce a split between the bulk of the profession and the educators. You can professionalize training too much and lose touch with the realities of community-based primary care.*

Meeke: *Surely you're not worried about the ivory tower idea. Wouldn't academic recognition be a good thing?*

Best: *I'm not worried about ivory towers as long as they've got solid foundations on earth and rock. But I am aware of the level of scepticism that exists among many GPs about the college circles, the regional hierarchies and GP academics. Much of it is false. But there is a danger of the patient-centred GP becoming self-centred. Academic ambitions can easily lead to a career-building, part-time GP. I like to think that any GP can become a trainer, a course organizer, a member of a representative committee. I would hate to see the day when the only way to contribute to training was by coming up through a single academically oriented channel like the university, where you couldn't get started without extra paper qualifications.*

Meeke: *Yes, I suppose that could mean that GPs like me in small-town practice wouldn't get a look in. There was a lot of speculation about the reasons for falling trainee numbers and the effects of this on small, vocational training schemes. The problems of one course organizer looking after all trainees in a district, including SHOs, and doing a lot more assessment point towards centralizing schemes on larger units with teams of course organizers. Each could become a sort of specialist in different aspects of vocational training.*

Best: *This reminds me of the change from single-handed practices to groups in health centres. Villages lost their doctor and the homely surgery gave way to intimidating large health centres. A lot was lost, but new possibilities opened up. I hope there will always be room for the small local outfit just as there is still room for the small practice. The link is technology. Properly equipped, the small organization can do nearly everything the large one can – and perhaps more efficiently. I'm too old to get to grips at this stage with creating databases, spread-sheets and surfing the Net. But distance now is no problem. I'm told you could run sub-regional offices from all the training centres through teleconferencing and e-mail links. Was there much talk about how new technology could help vocational training?*

Meeke: *Not a lot. There were some computer-based, self-assessment and teaching programmes mentioned, and an Internet demonstration. Lots of course organizers don't seem to have decent secretarial back-up, not to mention fax machines or word processors. I suppose I'd better get to know the computer at the postgraduate centre some time. I'll need it if the length of vocational training is extended and we have to keep track of more individuals.*

Best: *What, longer vocational training? That'll be the day! I suppose it was talked about in the '70s. There was a plan for a five-year training programme – three years' general professional training and two years' higher professional training, just like in hospital specialist training, but it was quietly buried. There was something in the Calman report about resurrecting that idea, wasn't there?*

Meeke: *Yes. You know there is the general feeling that one practice year is not enough. Some places now have one and a half years in practice and a shorter period of hospital jobs, and that looks like becoming the general rule. There's one place in Ireland which has a four-year course including a year in community health. If the endpoint of vocational training becomes blurred and merges into continuing medical education, perhaps with a two-year probationary period of supervised practice, that would meet a lot of the criticisms about the current inadequacy of vocational training.*

Best: *Yes, but isn't that a bit unrealistic? Surely the trend in recent years has been to emphasize the endpoint, you know – more trainees doing the College exam and the introduction of the other test – what's it called? I thought COs were all for formative assessment, and now you have two exams to get round.*

Meeke: *It's still called the Summative Assessment (I don't think anybody has thought up a real name for it yet). It generated a lot of heat at the conference, the usual gripes – exam domination, use of resources – you know the list. Some thought it was not so bad. It provides a real alternative to the College exam, provides options, costs the trainee nothing. There were even some College examiners who thought it had done the MRCGP good by forcing the pace of change.*

Best: *What was the balance of opinion?*

Meeke: *After blowing off steam most thought that too much was made of it and that it will not last, that the MRCGP might assimilate it, perhaps as a Part I exam that enables you to practice while preparing for Part II at a later time, even after completing VT. That really would take pressure off the registrar year, but less people would end up completing the exam.*

Best: *Which brings us back to the idea of higher professional training or more practice-based training. I hear some are proposing to abolish the hospital-based training altogether. That will raise a few eyebrows in the regional office!*

Meeke: *I think that may be the general intention. If hospitals think they can rely on GP–SHOs to keep them afloat, and that we need their SHO jobs for our training, then the status quo is not threatened. But, if they know they might lose half their SHO power, they might take the job of training them more seriously.*

Best: *It's just a bluff, then?*

Meeke: *I think it's more than that. The feeling is that the future of GP training must be in the hands of GPs. The primary care-led NHS implies just that. The swing towards undergraduate teaching in the community fits with that too. The commercial pressures of trust status make the hospitals more service orientated, squeezing out the educational aspects. These are an added burden which they might be quite happy to dump. Then they could get on with their business plans and performance indicators.*

Best: *How's it going to work, then?*

Meeke: *Nobody's too clear about that yet. Calman suggests that hospitals should be more self-sufficient, relying less on transient labour than on specialist trainees and a more broadly-based specialist grade. GP training should be community-based and less hospital dependent. The hospital contribution should be focused, more in line with generalist training needs. This means that trainees should get into training practices as early as possible, find out what they need to know and get it through a system of 'electives'. Over the training period they build up their portfolio of experience. There will still be hospital-based components, but these will be selected by the learners as short attachments to specialist units or clinics.*

Best: *Does this not imply a huge bureaucratic structure. You are talking about providing a rounded, individualized, mentored programme!*

Meeke: *The CO's role will have to be expanded if we are to co-ordinate the overall direction as well as provide the day-release course. So will that of the trainers, naturally.*

Best: *It sounds like the CO will be like a fundholder GP. Is that wise? Remember, the fundholding model was not an unqualified success.*

Meeke: *There are increasing fundholding elements to course organizing as it is. But we're talking about a commissioning-based model. It may be that each VT scheme will turn into a training consortium, with COs and trainers exercising purchasing and providing powers. They would contract with the region to provide whatever number of integrated three-year programmes the region projects it will need. Then they purchase short stints in any relevant learning situation which lies beyond the capacity of the consortium to provide from within its own resources. I don't see how a region could provide such a programme from a centralized base.*

Best: *I suppose a lot of specialist resources lie within training practices now that many of them contract in specialist-run clinics on their own premises, which the trainees should attend. Then there are the in-house clinics for child development, women's health and diabetes, minor surgery etc. Certainly, a lot of what used to be learned in hospital can now be got in a large training practice... it might work.*

Meeke: *We might even find ourselves sending trainees off on day release to hospital!*

Best: *Now you're being sardonic! But if you bring in the problem-based learning idea, the trainee group could commission specialist input on an ad-hoc basis. Case-based learning could mean that the trainee would follow selected cases through the hospital process. These problems and cases are included in his learning portfolio, which would later form the basis of assessed work. But it's bound to throw up problems like administration and financing.*

Meeke: *That's where the discussion groups at the course got a bit quiet, and started to talk about the good old days when being a course organizer meant organizing a course, once a week. Some came up with grandiose ideas about the GP training consortium financing all this through contracts with medical faculties for teaching students, with local GPs for providing programmes of CME, and hospital trusts for providing some of their specialist trainees' needs.*

Best: *Which brings us back to the earlier idea of the generic GP teacher – it doesn't need to be an individual; the consortium should have generic potential. But what would it offer the hospital? They haven't ever shown the slightest wish to have GPs as teachers.*

Meeke: *This is where we go back to Calman and general professional training. There is a strong recommendation, shared by the JCPTGP, that most clinicians need some experience in general practice during training, especially the more community-oriented specialisms.*

Best: *Yes... yes... so the training practices would take in their specialist trainees for a few months each while they provide specific learning situations for your registrars. It reminds me of the street economy during the 'hungry thirties' when the men were*

unemployed and the women earned a bit by taking in each others' washing to do...
economically neutral in theory, but does it work in practice?

Meeke: *There are all sorts of imponderables, of course. For a start it would make everyone*
put a proper price on training activities, properly value them, that is. It would use
the excess training capacity in general practice and it would be good for the profes-
sion as a whole. A lot of what GPs can teach would make useful packages for hospital
doctors – all that staff about consultation and communication skills, working in
small groups, how to make decisions about priorities on the basis of the community
denominator which would give them a realistic view of what problems are common
and important in practice.

Best: *Hey, slow up... you're getting beyond me with all this denominator stuff! Will all*
of this not collapse unless you solve the recruitment crisis? What's going to become
of your fancy consortium if you haven't any trainees?

Meeke: *I suppose if we are short of trainees we can still keep our trainers busy with pro-*
viding training for the hospitals and CME for GPs. Anyway, a lot of people feel that
the recruitment crisis has peaked – that it was the 1990 contract and the newness of
fundholding that scared off a lot of people, and all that will settle down. Besides,
setting out an attractive shop window by getting proper GP education through to
young doctors before they get embedded in the hospital mould could reverse the
process. Then we might be in a better place to offer a credible basis for higher profes-
sional training. At first this would have to be optional, with electives in public
health, research methods, a dissertation towards a Master's Degree, proper manage-
ment training and, maybe, overseas experience – all the sort of things that stimulate
and attract young people at present to hospital careers. We could, once again, attract
the brightest and best.

Best: *I like the bit about attracting the Best. I am almost tempted to come out of retirement*
and run with it. But it sounds like there was a bit of wine tasting going on at the
course. I hope that in the midst of all this speculation about the future there was
something about concrete, here-and-now issues, like what is happening for SHO
trainees, for instance?

Meeke: *A bit. Nothing very definite and a lot of people were concerned that not enough is*
happening there. Apparently there's a lot of militant SHOs around, but they get less
militant when they become registrars in practices. That leaves the next lot of SHOs
to get angry in turn, and there's not much change. However, some of them are get-
ting really good teaching now with the increase of block-release teaching schemes.
There's more attention being paid to integrated general professional training for all
junior doctors in the hospitals. A lot of people hope this will raise standards across
the board and relieve some of the pressure on the GP training curriculum. Another
controversial area was teaching about management. Most felt that it was important
to get a balance between the business and the human aspects of management.

Best: *I'm glad to hear that. Sometimes I think the government is trying to turn us into*
civil servants and accountants to run the health service for them. That changes the
training agenda. I've felt in recent years that the changes in health care delivery

have raised training issues which were in danger of marginalizing clinical medicine and the pastoral side of general practice. The growth points a few years ago were counselling and the time-consuming caring aspect. The paradox is that the old primary care team which we used to talk about so much is being taken apart, yet there is more and more talk about interdisciplinary training.

Meeke: *I didn't hear much said about that at the conference. The other disciplines are becoming so autonomous that it's hard to see how to develop that in vocational training.*

Best: *It will probably be more a feature of continuing medical education. I hear they're beginning to call it CPD – continuing professional development. In my day CPD was an obstetric crisis when the head got too big to deliver! But, like everything else in continuing medical education it's got to start somewhere – that means vocational training, even perhaps the undergraduate curriculum. What else was being talked about?*

Meeke: *It's hard to remember, there was so much – everybody in groups and huddles between sessions blazing away about everything under the sun – how to include sessions in the course on the needs of adolescents and all the transcultural implications of training for practice in a cosmopolitan society; the growth in demand for complementary medicine; the manpower implications of a united Europe. There is a real influx of trainees from other EU states. They have special training needs. Many of our fellow Europeans seem to have quite different traditions of medical practice. One or two people were very interested in the growth of primary care in Eastern Europe and 'Third World' countries. It seems we have something to learn from them about appropriate technology and health care delivery – use of paramedics and nurse practitioners, for example – and that we should be doing more to help them in developing primary care teaching programmes.*

Best: *Yes, we can't let differences in systems of care blind us to the fundamental similarities of training for health care everywhere. Quite a lot of course organizers have been invited to visit and advise on training in other countries. So, do you feel your first year has broadened your horizons?*

Meeke: *At an alarming rate. I've got to remember that I'm still a full-time GP. The real development next year will be to make sure that the business of course organizing feeds something into how my practice is developing rather than diverting energy from it.*

Best: *That's important. I've just thought of a new acronym for your collection – BPDCO (Balanced Professional Development for Course Organizers). One more thing...*

Meeke: *That's not an acronym, that's an abbreviation! Here's a real acronym. It will be the name of an organization I might set up to retail training techniques to hospitals. It's called SALARIED, the Syndicate of Advisers in Learning, Assessment and Research in Educational Development!*

Best: *I like that. What I was going to say a moment ago was that I've been getting the feeling that you're ahead of me. I'm enjoying our sessions more and more. At the start I felt I was supporting you in coping. Now I feel I am learning more from you than you are from me. I'm not saying we should stop having these sessions – there is plenty still to talk about. Now it's not the problems of survival, but the problems of growth. I hope you'll still drop round for a glass and keep me up-to-date on developments. For now I think it's time to break a bottle of champagne across your bow and declare you well and truly launched. And don't think you're going to have the last word. I've just thought of an acronym for your syndicate – The Innovation Co-operative for Medical Education. In short, INCOME.*

Bibliography

Chapter 1

McEvoy PJ (1993) The new course organizer: problems, anxieties and needs. *Postgraduate Education for General Practice.* **4**: 55–9.

Chapter 2

Squires G (1994) *A new model of teaching and training.* Published by the author, Geoffrey Squires, 186 Victoria Avenue, Hull HU5 3DY.

Toon PD, Suckling H and Lawrie J (1995) What is the half-day release for? *Education for General Practice.* **6**(2): 171–4.

Chapter 3

ACO (1997) *Minutes of the Annual General Meeting.* ACO, Ripon.

Calman K (1995) *Hospital doctors: training for the future. Supplementary reports.* NHS Executive, Leeds.

Evans S (1990) The work of the course organizer. *Postgraduate Education for General Practice.* **1**: 112–14.

Fairclough D (1985) Outline job description of a course organizer. *J Assoc Course Organizers.* **1**: 23–8.

Lewis AP (1986) Report on course organizers' timesheet questionnaire. *J Assoc Course Organizers.* **1**: 137–45.

Percy D and Pitts J (1994) The purchaser and provider split in general practice education. *Education for General Practice.* **5**: 229–33.

Pereira Gray DJ (1986) Preface. In: *Course organizers in general practice. Occasional Paper 34.* RCGP, London.

RCGP (1989) *An educational strategy for the '90s.* RCGP, London.

Styles R (1986) Inter-regional peer-group visiting of vocational training scheme. *J Assoc Course Organizers.* **2**: 86–90.

Williams AH (1986) *Course organizers in general practice. Occasional Paper 34.* RCGP, London.

Chapter 4

Brookfield SD (1986) *Understanding and facilitating adult learning.* Open University Press, Milton Keynes.

Curry L (1983) An organization of learning styles: theory and constraints. *Eric Document.* **275**: 185.

Hayden J (1996) Developing vocational training for British general practice – a system for the future. *Education for General Practice.* **7**: 1–7.

Honey P and Mumford A (1986) *The manual of learning styles.* Peter Honey, Maidenhead.

McEvoy P (1992) Core educational beliefs. *Postgraduate Education for General Practice.* **3**: 232.

Myers IB (1962) *The Myers–Briggs type indicator manual.* Educational Testing Service, Princeton.

Neighbour R (1990) Icarus and Daedelus: myths, methods and motivation in vocational training. *Postgraduate Education for General Practice.* **1**: 165–73.

Newble D and Clarke RM (1986) The approaches to learning of students in a traditional and in an innovative problem-based medical school. *Medical Education.* **20**: 267–73.

Newble D and Entwhistle NJ (1986) Learning styles and approaches: implications for medical education. *Medical Education.* **20**: 162–75.

Riding R and Cheema I (1991) Cognitive styles: an overview and integration. *Educational Psychology.* **11**: 193–215.

Rogers A (1988) *Teaching adults.* Open University Press, Milton Keynes.

Schön DA (1983) *The reflective practitioner.* Temple Smith, London.

SCPME (1991) *Learning general practice.* Scottish Council for Postgraduate Medical Education, Edinburgh.

Stott NC (1979) The exceptional potential of each general practice consultation. *JRCGP.* **29**: 201–15.

Chapter 5

RCGP (1990) *Educational strategy for the '90s.* RCGP, London.

RCGP (1994) *Portfolio-based learning in general practice. Occasional Paper 63.* RCGP, London.

RCGP (1996) *Significant event auditing. Occasional Paper 70.* RCGP, London.

Tripps D (1993) *Critical events in teaching: developing professional judgement.* Routledge, London.

Chapter 6

Bahrami J (1989) Who is assessing course organizers? *J Assoc Course Organizers.* **4**: 130–2.

Ball C and Siegel S (1995) Course organizer assessment – the West Midlands approach. *Education for General Practice.* **6**(3): 230–2.

Bligh J (1993) The S-SDLRS: a short questionnaire about self-directed learning. *Postgraduate Education for General Practice.* **4**(2): 121–5.

Brooks D (1986) Assessment – the course organizer's role. *Postgraduate Education for General Practice.* **2**: 13–17.

Crabbe I (1986) Annual reports and inter-course comparison. *Postgraduate Education for General Practice.* **2**: 72–4.

Field S (1995) The use of video recording in general practice education. *Education for General Practice.* **6**(1): 49–58.

Gambril E *et al.* (1991) *Vocational training working group – assessment of trainees.* RCGP, London.

Gibbs G *et al.* (1988) *53 interesting ways to appraise your teaching.* Technical and Educational Services, Bristol.

Gronlund NA (1988) *Stating objectives for classroom instruction* (2nd edn). Macmillan, New York.

Hayden J (1996) Developing vocational training for British general practice – a system for the future. *Education for General Practice.* **7**(1): 1–7.

Honey P and Mumford A (1992) *The manual of learning styles.* Peter Honey, Maidenhead.

JCPTGP (1992) *Guidelines on formative assessment.* Joint Committee on Postgraduate Education for General Practice, London.

JCPTGP (1995) *Summative assessment in vocational training for general practice – first position paper.* Joint Committee on Postgraduate Training for General Practice, London.

Merrison AW (1975) *The Merrison Committee Report.* HMSO, London.

Newble DJ and Entwhistle NJ (1986) Learning styles and approaches: implications for medical education. *Medical Education.* **20**: 162–75.

RCGP (1988) *Rating scales for vocational training in general practice. Occasional Paper 40.* RCGP, London.

RCP (1997) *A core curriculum for senior house officers in general (internal) medicine and the medical specialties.* Royal College of Physicians, London.

Sackin P *et al.* (1988) Trainee-centred assessment. ACO working party report. *J Assoc Course Organizers.* **4**: 37–51.

Styles R (1986) Inter-regional peer-group visiting of vocational training scheme. *Postgraduate Education for General Practice.* **2**: 86–90.

Tait I (1987) Agreed educational objectives for the hospital period of vocational training. *J Assoc Course Organizers.* **2**(3): 179–82.

Chapter 7

ACO (1997) *Minutes of the 1997 annual general meeting.* ACO, Ripon.

Calman K (1995) *Hospital doctors: training for the future. Supplementary reports.* NHS Management Executive, Leeds.

Lindsay P *et al.* (1996) *Pass summative assessment and the MRCGP.* Saunders, London.

JCPTGP (1987) *Assessment and vocational training for general practice: final report of a JCPTGP working party.* Joint Committee on Postgraduate Education for General Practice, London.

JCPTGP (1992) *Interim report of the working party on assessment.* Joint Committee on Postgraduate Education for General Practice, London.

JCPTGP (1993) *Report of the summative assessment working party.* Joint Committee on Postgraduate Education for General Practice, London.

JCPTGP (1995) *Summative assessment of vocational training in general practice.* Joint Committee on Postgraduate Education for General Practice, London.

RCGP (1985) *What sort of doctor?* Royal College of General Practitioners, London.

Chapter 8

Bligh J (1995) Problem-based learning in medicine: an introduction. *Postgraduate Medical Journal.* **71**: 323–6.

Cross KP (1975) Learner-centred curricula. In: Vermilye DW (ed) *Learner-centred reform.* Jossey-Bass, Oxford.

Editorial (1986) Carrousel courses. *J Assoc Course Organizers.* **1**: 43.

Engel C (1992) Problem-based learning. *British Journal of Hospital Medicine.* **48**(6): 325–9.

Ferrier B (1990) Problem-based learning: does it make a difference? *Journal of Dental Education.* **54**(9): 550–1.

Freire P (1972) *Pedagogy of the oppressed and cultural action for freedom.* Penguin, Harmondsworth.

GMC Training Committee (1987) *Recommendations on the training of specialists.* General Medical Council, London.

GMSC (1996) *Defining core services in general practice: reclaiming professional control.* British Medical Association, London.

Gronlund A (1978) *Stating objectives for classroom instruction.* Macmillan, New York.

JCPTGP (1997) *Recommendations to regions on the selection and re-selection of hospital posts (draft).* Joint Committee on Postgraduate Training for General Practice, London.

McEvoy P (1995) Vocational training for general practice: the UK story. *Annals of Community-oriented Education.* **8**: 127–36.

Neighbour R (1996) *The inner apprentice.* Petroc, Newbury.

Newble DI and Clarke RM (1986) The approaches to learning of students in a traditional and in an innovative problem-based medical school. *Medical Education.* **20**: 267–73.

RCGP (1988) *Priority objectives for vocational training. Occasional Paper 30 (2nd edn).* RCGP, London.

RCGP (1989) *Rating scales for vocational training in general practice. Occasional Paper 40.* RCGP, London.

RCGP (1990) *An educational strategy for the '90s.* RCGP, London.

RCP (1997) *A core curriculum for senior house officers in general (internal) medicine and the medical specialties.* Royal College of Physicians, London.

Rogers A (1986) *Teaching adults.* Open University Press, Milton Keynes.

Salmon E and Savage R (1997) A professional development year in general practice: the vocationally trained associate scheme. *Education for General Practice.* **8**: 112–20.

Samuel O (1990a) *Towards a curriculum for general practice training. Occasional Paper 44.* RCGP, London.

Samuel O (1990b) What should trainees learn? *Postgraduate Education for General Practice.* **1**: 160–4.

Schön DA (1983) *The reflective practitioner.* Temple Smith, London.

Seiler R (1986) Letter to the Editor *J Assoc Course Organizers.* **1**: 135.

Tait I (1987) Agreed educational aims for the hospital period of vocational training. *J Assoc Course Organizers.* **3**: 179–81.

Weston J (1986) Around the courses. *J Assoc Course Organizers.* **2**: 45–7.

Woodward CA (1989) The effects of the innovations in medical education at McMaster: a report of follow-up studies. *MEDUCS.* **2**(3): 64–8.

Chapter 9

Gau D (1994) Decision theory: the logic for general practice in the nineties. In: *Members' Reference Book 1994.* Royal College of General Practitioners, London.

Honey P and Mumford A (1992) *A manual of learning style.* Peter Honey, Maidenhead.

McEvoy PJ (1975) The mortality committee as an educational and administrative tool. *Lancet.* **25**: 210–14.

McEvoy PJ (1997) Continuing medical education in general practice: the UK story. *Education for Health.* **10**(2): 221–33.

Myers IB (1962) *The Myers–Briggs type indicator manual.* Educational Testing Service, Princeton.

Neighbour R (1987) *The inner consultation.* Kluwer Academic, London.

O'Donnell M (1986) The teaching game. In: *Doctor, doctor: the insider's guide to the games doctors play.* Gollancz, London.

Pringle M (1995) *Significant event auditing. Occasional Paper 70.* RCGP, London.

Prochaska JO and di Clemente CR (1986) Towards a comprehensive model of change. In: *Treating addictive behaviors: processes of change.* Miller RW and Heather N (eds). Plenum Press, New York.

Riding R (1994) *Personal styles awareness and personal development.* Learning and Training Technology, Birmingham.

Schön D (1983) *The reflective practitioner.* Temple Smith, London.

Squires D (1994) *A new model of teaching and training.* Published by the author, Geoffrey Squires, 186 Victoria Avenue, Hull HU5 3DY.

Wilson DJ (1988) The invaluable art of unlearning. *Journal of the Royal Society of Medicine.* **83**: 3–6.

Chapter 10

Hopson B and Scally M (1981) *Life skill teaching.* McGraw-Hill, London

Kindred M (1995) *Once upon a group.* Available from the author, 20 Dover Street, Southwell, Nottingham NG25 0EZ.

Chapter 11

Hopson B and Scally M (1981) *Life skills teaching.* McGraw-Hill, London.

Tuckman BW (1965) Developmental sequences in small groups. *Psychological Bulletin.* **63**: 384–99.

Chapter 12

Calman K (1993) *Hospital doctors: training for the future.* NHS Executive, Leeds.

Calman K (1995) *Hospital doctors: training for the future. Supplementary reports.* NHS Executive, Leeds.

Dillner L (1993) Senior house officers: the lost tribes. *BMJ.* **307**: 1149–51.

GMSC (1996) *Study leave for GP registrars, prepared by the GMSC GP registrars' subcommittee, August 1996.* British Medical Association, London.

Hand C (1994) Joint hospital visiting: problems and solutions. *Education for General Practice.* 5(3): 247–53.

Hayden J (1996) Developing vocational training for British general practice. *Education for General Practice.* 7: 1–7.

JCPTGP (1996) *Recommendations to regions on the selection and reselection of hospital posts.* Joint Committee on Postgraduate Training for General Practice, London.

Kearley K (1990) An evaluation of the hospital component of general practice vocational training. *British Journal of General Practice.* 40: 409–14.

Kelly D and Murray TS (1997) An assessment of hospital training for general practice in the West of Scotland. *Education for General Practice.* 8(3): 220–6.

Orme-Smith A (1997) *A new look at general practice vocation training.* Minutes of the 1997 Annual General Meeting of the Association of Course Organizers.

RCGP (1988) *Oxford regional course organisers and regional advisers group. Priority objectives for general practice vocational training.* Royal College of General Practitioners, London.

RCGP (1993) *The quality of hospital-based education for general practice.* Royal College of General Practitioners, London.

RCGP (1994a) *Members' yearbook 1994.* Royal College of General Practitioners, London.

RCGP (1994b) *Education and training for general practice. Policy statement 3.* Royal College of General Practitioners, London.

RCP (1997) *A core curriculum for senior house officers in general (internal) medicine and the medicine specialities* (2nd edn). Royal College of Physicians, London.

Savage R *et al.* (1996) Registrar training for general practice: a pilot study of 18 months of hospital posts and 18 months in general practice. *Education of General Practice.* 7(3): 191–8.

Savage R *et al.* (1997) Vocational training for general practice: course organiser controlled funding to construct innovative SHO posts. *Education for General Practice.* 8(4): 280–7.

SCOPME (1991) *Improving the experience.* Standing Committee on Postgraduate Medical Education, London.

Styles E *et al.* (1993) The hospital component of vocational training for general practice: the views of course organisers. *Postgraduate Education for General Practice.* 4(3): 203–8.

Styles W (1990) But what now? Some unresolved problems of training for general practice. The William Pickles Lecture. *British Journal of General Practice.* 40: 270–6.

Tait I (1987) Agreed educational objectives for the hospital period of vocational training. *J Assoc Course Organizers.* 3: 179–81.

Torry R (1996) The training needs of hospital general practice registrars in SE Thames. *Education for General Practice.* 7: 221–8.

WHO (1995) *A charter for general practice/family medicine in Europe.* World Health Organization, Regional Office for Europe, Copenhagen.

Chapter 13

Belbin RM (1991) *Management teams, why they succeed or fail.* Heinemann, London.

Burke RJ (1971) Are you fed up with work? *Personnel Administration (US).* Jan–Feb.

Dunham J (1988) Time and work management. In: McDerment L *Stress care.* Social Care Association (Education), Surrey.

Ends E and Page CW (1977) *Organisational teambuilding.* University Press of America, London.

Fox RD, Mazmanian PE and Putnam RW (1989) *Changing and learning in the lives of physicians.* Praeger, London.

Francis D and Young D (1979) *Improving work groups: a practical manual for teambuilding.* University Associates Inc, Mansfield.

GMC (1995) *Duties of a doctor: guidance from the General Medical Council.* GMC, London.

Hayden J (1996) Developing vocational training in British general practice – a system for the future. *Education for General Practice.* **7**: 1–7.

ICGP (1991) Time management: key ideas. In: *Handbook and diary.* Irish College of General Practitioners, Dublin.

Irvine D and Irvine S (1997) *Making sense of audit* (2nd edn). Radcliffe Medical Press, Oxford.

Jones RVH (1996) *Working together, learning together.* Occasional Paper 33. RCGP, London.

Kindred M and Goldsmith M (1997) *Communicating with the public.* 4M Publications (20 Dover Street, Southwell, Nottinghamshire NG25 0EZ).

McDerment L (1988) *Stress care.* Social Care Association (Education), Surrey.

Neighbour R (1996) *The inner apprentice.* Petroc Press, Newbury.

Norman GR and Schmidt HG (1992) The psychological basis of problem-based learning: a review of the evidence. *Academic Medicine.* **67**(9): 557–65.

Oxley J (1997) Appraising doctors and dentists in training. *BMJ* (Classified). **1 Nov**: 2–3.

Pines A and Maslach C (1978) Characteristics of staff burnout in mental health settings. *Hospital and Community Psychiatry.* **29**: 233–7.

Pollar O (1993) *Get organised.* Kogan Page, London.

RCGP (1988) *Rating scales for vocational training in general practice.* Occasional Paper 40. Royal College of General Practitioners, London.

RCGP (1989) *Priority objectives for vocational training.* Occasional Paper 30. Royal College of General Practitioners, London.

Samuel O (1987) Management is about people. *J Assoc Course Organizers*. **3**: 34.

Sargent A and Wilkinson A (1980) *Decision taking, guidance on getting decisions taken and achieving co-operation*. Industrial Society, London.

Schön D (1983) *The reflective practitioner*. Temple Smith, London.

SCOPME (1991) *Improving the experience*. Standing Committee on Postgraduate Medical Education, London.

SCOPME (1997) *Multiprofessional working and learning: sharing the educational challenge*. SCOPME, London.

Shapiro JB and Clawson TW (1982) Stress and anxiety management. (Paper presented at the Annual Meeting of the American Association for Counselling and Development European Branch, Munich.) Quoted in McDerment L (1988) *Stress care*. Social Care Association (Education), Surrey.

Tate P (1997) *The doctors' communication handbook* (2nd edn). Radcliffe Medical Press, Oxford.

Woodcock M (1979) *Teamwork development*. Gower, London.

Chapter 14

Coles C (1990) Making audit truly educational. *Postgraduate Medical Journal*. **66**(Suppl 3): S32–6.

Collins PA (1997) *Teleworking*. MBA Thesis, University of Ulster, Jordanstown.

Mant D (1998) R&D in primary care – an NHS priority (editorial). *British Journal of General Practice*. **48**: 426, 871.

McWhinney JB (1989) The need for a transformed clinical method. In: Stewart M and Roter D (eds) *Communicating with medical patients*. Sage, London.

Macauley D (1994) READER: an acronym to aid critical reading by general practitioners. *British Journal of General Practice*. **44**: 83–5.

MRC (1997) *Primary health care* [topic review]. Medical Research Council, London.

Moran IB (1990) A guide to project assessment. *Horizons*. **August**: 457.

Pereira Gray D (1991) Research in general practice, the law of inverse opportunity. *British Medical Journal*. **302**: 1380–2.

Pollar O (1993) *Get organised*. Kogan Page, London.

Radda G (1998) Primary care research: the MRC's proposals (Editorial). *British Journal of General Practice*. **48**: 426, 872.

RCGP (1988) *Trainee projects. Occasional Paper 29*. Royal College of General Practitioners, London.

Rowan J and Reason P (1981) On making sense. In: Reason P and Rowan J (eds) *Human inquiry: a source book for new paradigm research*. John Wiley, Chichester.

Chapter 15

Calman K (1995) *Hospital doctors: training for the future.* A supplementary report by the Working Group Commissioners to consider the implications for general medical practice arising from the principal report. Department of Health, London.

Garrett T (1992) Personal communication.

JCPTGP (1992*a*) *Recommendations to regions for the establishment of criteria for the approval and reapproval of trainers in general practice.* Joint Committee on Postgraduate Training for General Practice, London.

JCPTGP (1992*b*) *Accreditation of regions and schemes for vocational training in general practice: (1) General guidance; (2) Guidance for visitors and regional advisers.* Joint Committee on Postgraduate Training for General Practice, London.

JCPTGP (1997) *Recommendations to regions for selection and re-selection of hospital posts.* Joint Committee on Postgraduate Training for General Practice, London.

NHS (1997) *The National Health Service (Vocational Training for General Medical Practice) Regulations 1997.* The Stationery Office Ltd, London.

NHS Management Executive (1991) *Working for patients: postgraduate medical and dental education.* Department of Health, London.

Orme-Smith A (1993) A new genus: a working paper for discussion. *Postgraduate Education for General Practice.* **4**: 69–71.

Terry J (1991) Personal communication.

Chapter 17

Boerma WGW, de Jong FA and Mulder PH (1993) *Health care and general practice around Europe.* Netherlands Institute of Primary Health Care, Utrecht.

Buckley G and Heyrmann J (1994) Europe and training for general practice (editorial). *Education for General Practice,* **5**: 241–5.

King M (1966) *Medical care in developing countries.* Oxford University Press, Oxford.

Kinworth A (1994) Where there is no general practitioner: training for family medicine in Latvia. *Education for General Practice.* **5**: 288–93.

Lember M (1996) Family practice training in Estonia. *International Family Medicine.* **28**: 282–6.

Sips F (1995) A common basis for general practice/family medicine in Europe. *Journal of Family Practice.* **41**(1): 24–6.

Index